expect a *Miracle*

expect a *Miracle*

Unwavering faith through fetal surgery

andrea merkord

TATE PUBLISHING & *Enterprises*

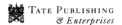

TATE PUBLISHING
 & *Enterprises*

Tate Publishing is committed to excellence in the publishing industry. Our staff of highly trained professionals, including editors, graphic designers, and marketing personnel, work together to produce the very finest books available. The company reflects the philosophy established by the founders, based on Psalms 68:11,

"THE LORD GAVE THE WORD AND GREAT WAS THE COMPANY OF THOSE WHO PUBLISHED IT."

If you would like further information, please contact us:
1.888.361.9473 | www.tatepublishing.com
TATE PUBLISHING & *Enterprises*, LLC | 127 E. Trade Center Terrace
Mustang, Oklahoma 73064 USA

*Expect A Miracle*
Copyright © 2007 by Andrea Merkord. All rights reserved.

This title is also available as a Tate Out Loud product.
Visit www.tatepublishing.com for more information

No part of this publication may be reproduced, stored in a retrieval system or transmitted in any way by any means, electronic, mechanical, photocopy, recording or otherwise without the prior permission of the author except as provided by USA copyright law.

Scripture quotations marked "NIV" are taken from the *Holy Bible, New International Version* ®, Copyright © 1973, 1978, 1984 by International Bible Society. Used by permission of Zondervan Publishing House. All rights reserved.

Scripture quotations marked "TLB" are taken from *The Living Bible* / Kenneth N. Taylor: Tyndale House, © Copyright 1997, 1971 by Tyndale House Publishers, Inc. Used by permission. All rights reserved.

Names, descriptions, entities, and incidents included in the story are based on the lives of real people.

Book design copyright © 2007 by Tate Publishing, LLC. All rights reserved.
*Cover design by Lindsay B. Behrens*
*Interior design by Leah LeFlore*

Published in the United States of America

ISBN: 978-1-6024707-7-4

07.03.26

# DEDICATION

*For William and Andrew, who I see every day in the twinkle of Thomas's sparkling blue eyes. Thomas, you provide more laughter and joy than I could have ever imagined.*

# ACKNOWLEDGEMENTS

Thank you to my Lord and Savior, Jesus Christ, who gave me the motivation to write a book without any knowledge of where it would lead. Sean, you are my perfect match. Sometimes we wonder exactly where that match was made, but aren't we a pair? We'll see where the next fifty years takes us. It ought to be an exciting ride! Tate Publishing, thank you for your vision and willingness to put your resources into my story. Eileene Werner and Jennie Lamme, thank you for your enthusiastic participation in reading through my first drafts. Your ideas were invaluable. Thanks go to my family for their support: Tony and Carol Merkord, Steve and Mary Chenault, Craig and Tandi Merkord, Amber Chenault, April Bays, and Karla Hughes. A special thank you to Mark and Marcy Wellman, who helped build the rock solid foundation that my firm faith stands on today. Without John Granby, those nine months would have been even worse than they already were. God used you, buddy, willingly or not! Love ya!

# CONTENTS

FOREWORD                                    11

*1* STRENGTH FOR FEAR                       12

*2* THE DARK SIDE OF JOY                     38

*3* PEACE FOR DESPAIR                        66

*4* GLADNESS FOR MOURNING                    98

*5* GARDETTO'S, ANYONE?                     123

*6* BEAUTY FOR ASHES                        151

*7* A PROMISE KEPT                          173

# THE SAGA OF MERKORD

*foreword*

Some things don't come easy. The personal reflections of Andrea Merkord about the incredible saga she went through to have a healthy and thriving boy certainly illustrate how difficult it can be for a mother and her family to give their baby a chance at life. Her personal experience and emotional reaction to what seemed, at the time, to be a series of incredibly unfair catastrophes for her pregnancy is indeed moving. Her story speaks volumes about her determination to give her boy every chance despite the fact that it meant considerable risk to her. Remember that she did not herself have a threatening medical problem but had to share the risk of the intervention to help her fetus. This story also sheds light on how very difficult it is to go through this ordeal.

There is another aspect to this story. It makes us appreciate the contribution of heroic mothers and families to the advancement of knowledge that directly contributes to advances in treatment for other children and subsequent generations. These families essentially volunteer not only to help their fetus but also to contribute knowledge that will impact other families in the future. Their sacrifice and struggle contribute directly to advancement of fetal therapy.

**Michael Harrison, MD**
Professor of Clinical Surgery, Pediatrics, Obstetrics, Gynecology and Reproductive Sciences, Emeritus
Founding Director, Fetal Treatment Center
University of California, San Francisco

# STRENGTH FOR FEAR

**PSALM 139:13-16 NIV**
For you created my inmost being; you knit me together in my mother's womb. I praise you because I am fearfully and wonderfully made; your works are wonderful, I know that full well. My frame was not hidden from you when I was made in the secret place. When I was woven together in the depths of the earth, Your eyes saw my unformed body. All the days ordained for me were written in your book before one of them came to be.

While Sean and Andrea sat in the ultrasound room at St. Charles hospital waiting to see those first images of the life inside of her, they were wondering if it really could be twins. They were told it was a real possibility and that's what they were there to find out, but the words spoken by the radiologist, Mimi, were the last thing they expected to hear. She immediately said, "Yep, there's two."

Andrea looked at Sean and smiled, but they quickly turned back to the screen to watch their babies. After scanning the area for a few more minutes in silence, Mimi said with uneasy breath, "Well, I see three heads, but only two bodies."

Andrea's eyes couldn't leave the screen, but her left hand reached out to the side where Sean sat in shock and found a place tucked in his much larger hand. Unable to process the information and the images she was seeing, Andrea let her mind think back to when she and Sean first decided they were ready to have children.

## MATTHEW 19:26 NIV

Jesus looked at them and said, "With man this is impossible, but with God all things are possible."

From the time they had gotten married, Sean and Andrea knew they wanted to wait until after they had been married for two years to have children. Everything had to be carefully planned in their perfectly timed lives. Andrea had always dreamed of a girl. She had two sisters and thought she was geared to have girls. She would never know what to do with a boy if she had one. When November came around, Andrea couldn't wait to start planning the future wee one. The bad thing was that they were planning a trip to Hawaii the following September and didn't want anything to interfere with that, so they decided to wait a couple of months longer. That way, if they got pregnant right out of the gate, they wouldn't be too far along in the pregnancy for Andrea to travel. By the end of January, the anticipation had reached its peak and Andrea could wait no longer. She threw away her pack of birth control pills (with Sean in agreement, of course!). Game on! Her logical side told her it could take a while to actually get pregnant, so she shouldn't get her hopes up of it happening immediately. A couple weeks later, her younger sister, April, called to chat and asked if they had started trying for a baby yet. Andrea told her, "Well, we haven't even gone a month yet."

April said, "Well, I beat you!"

"No way. I didn't even know you were trying," Andrea said in shocked surprise.

"Well, it happened the first month so we really didn't have time to tell anyone."

Secretly, Andrea was a little jealous but also excited because it would be so fun if they were pregnant at the same time. Now she really hoped it would happen right away.

expect a miracle  *13*

The end of March came with Andrea's twenty-eighth birthday staring her in the face. She and Sean drove a couple of hours over the beautiful Cascade Mountains of Oregon to spend the weekend with family. Saturday morning, Andrea went to spend some time with her old high school dance team buddy, Christina, who happened to live conveniently just around the corner from Andrea's parents. She was able to finally see Christina's five-month-old boy, James. Andrea told her it was the second month of trying for a baby, and she should know that weekend if they weren't pregnant yet.

Christina could barely contain herself and ran with girlish glee to her bathroom to grab a pregnancy test that she had hidden away. Andrea didn't even want to take it. She assumed the test would be negative even if she was pregnant because it was just too early to tell yet. It would only be a let down to take a test too soon, if one has no inclination that she might actually be pregnant.

Andrea was resting in a recliner when Christina animatedly brought the test over, instructions in hand, and positioned it deviously on the arm of the chair next to her, stating, "I'll just leave this here in case you change your mind."

With that, she smugly returned to the kitchen to make James some food. The curiosity was killing Andrea, and she finally hollered, "Fine!" and ran into the bathroom giggling.

She immediately cried out, "There's a line!"

Christina jumped and screamed so loudly that she startled James, who began to cry. She ran to the bathroom and Andrea showed her the test. Christina said, "You ding dong! There's always one line! You have to wait and see if there are two lines."

Andrea was disappointed. They left the test in the bathroom and waited the instructed five minutes before looking again. After the seemingly eternal five minute wait, they looked again, and, lo and behold, there was a faint second line. Andrea didn't want to get excited because she wasn't sure it was a positive result. Christina was certain it was positive.

They had a lunch date in Salem with Andrea's mom and two sisters to celebrate Andrea's birthday, and it was almost time to hit the road. Andrea wanted to go show her mom the pregnancy test if they could catch her before she left home. Mary was just getting ready to leave her house for the lunch date when the two girls came to the door bursting with excitement.

Andrea whipped out the pregnancy test, which she had cautiously placed in a sealed plastic bag. Mary looked at her and questioned, "What?"

Andrea told her the story of how Christina just *happened* to have a pregnancy test laying around, so she had taken it.

After they were seated at the Olive Garden restaurant in Salem, Amber, Andrea's older sister by two years, was the next to arrive, and Andrea told her the exciting news as well. Only halfway kidding, Amber said, "I'm so jealous. I want to be pregnant too."

April arrived shortly after getting off work at the vet clinic in Silverton, a small town just outside of Salem. She was still wearing her loose-fitting scrubs, but you could tell she was about ten weeks along in her own pregnancy and starting to fill out a little. When April came to the other side of the table to give Andrea her birthday gift, Andrea exchanged with her the plastic bag.

April smiled and said, "When did you find out?"

Andrea gave her the run down on how the morning had progressed. They hugged, and everyone was delighted. Andrea felt bad because everyone was finding out before Sean. However, she didn't want to call him and tell him over the phone either. It would just have to wait for the right moment.

expect a miracle *15*

When Andrea arrived back at Sean's parents' house in Albany, she pulled Sean aside by the hand to his old bedroom. Without saying a word, she jumped onto the bed, held the test up between them, and just grinned, waiting for his response. He got a teasing smirk on his face and said, "I don't think so. I'm not ready."

Shortly after that, they were in the dining room with Sean's parents having a barbeque dinner. Sean, who was concealing his excitement said, "Andrea has something to tell you guys."

Andrea turned to Sean and told them it was he who had something to share with them. He refused to tell, so it was left to Andrea. So she spit it out.

"We had a positive pregnancy test today."

They were taken by complete surprise. After dinner, Andrea drove into town to get another pregnancy test that she could take first thing in the morning. She awoke early to use the restroom and carried the bag in with her very quietly. After quietly shutting the door and turning on the light, she proceeded to take the test and wait another agonizing five minutes for the results. After five minutes of eye rolling, thumb twiddling, and clock watching, she dared to look at the test. This time that second line was just a little darker. She was convinced now and hurriedly crawled back in bed to tell Sean it was true. They were pregnant!

They spent the day on Sunday enjoying the sunny, but cool weather and calling different family members to share the good news. When Monday came and they returned to work, Andrea was bursting at the seams to tell Trisha, who would share in her excitement. Andrea, Trisha, and Elizabeth had big smiles from ear to ear when the owner, John, came in and he guessed, "You're PG?"

He could read her excitement and was happy for her too. John had always made sure the atmosphere at his optical lab was light and fun, while productive. It was the craziest place at which most of them had ever worked. He told inappropriate jokes to every person who walked in the door, some of whom weren't quite sure how to take him. Trisha fit quite well with his laid back nature. She was a pretty, young, fun-loving girl, who was great with the customers, and everyone liked her. Her small features and mischievous smile were often hidden behind hair that was thick like a horse's mane, brown, and half-way down her back with the ends always neatly curled under, along with a thick row of bangs curled down her forehead. Her personality was a magnet to anyone who met her.

John couldn't figure out how these two opposite people could become such good friends. There were a couple of months when Trisha and Andrea were buried with work in the office by themselves doing the work of four people. They had recently lost two other office personnel. They worked well together and were forced to get to know each other in a flash. They were both hard workers and could cover each other in any of the job duties of the front office, which worked to their advantage. After a while, they started getting together outside of work.

Trisha would go to Andrea's house in the morning before work and they would do Tae-Bo workout videos downstairs in the living room. Neither Andrea nor Trisha had any business being seen before showers and make-up, which made them laugh at each other every morning. After their workout, Andrea would go upstairs to wake up Sean and hop in the shower, while Trisha would get ready in the downstairs bathroom. It was a tiny room with just a toilet to the left, and across from that, a sink to the right. There was a small dividing wall and just beyond that were the washer and dryer. There was usually some laundry running in the morning, and it gave Trisha a jolt all the time. The dryer had a buzzer on it to inform that

expect a miracle  *17*

the load was almost done. It alarmed three times about five minutes apart. Trisha usually had the door closed when it went off and swore she was going deaf because of it.

Trisha received a lot of flack at work because she was so easy to tease. Elizabeth was always quick on her toes with short retorts that usually weren't in Trisha's favor. With injured ego, Trisha would playfully turn her head up and look away, saying, "I'm not talking to you anymore today."

John had nicknamed Trisha, "Bob," because when she had first started working there, he had a hard time remembering her name. Everyone lovingly knew her as Bob. One morning, Bob was enjoying her favorite doughnut, the tasty, fluffy maple bar. She had left it on her desk and went out to the lab to find something. When she returned, it was gone. She yelled at Andrea accusingly, "Where's my maple bar?"

Andrea helped her look around, assuming John had hidden it somewhere.

She asked Bob, "Are you sure you didn't finish it?"

Trisha said, "Well, I guess I did," and they left it at that.

The next day, Trisha was helping a customer on the phone and went to pull a tray out of a pile of stackable plastic eyeglass trays. She picked up the tray she was looking for and immediately started laughing and yelling, "Angela!"

She called Andrea "Angela" because it had always made Andrea mad when people called for her and mistook her name for Angela. It became a running joke.

"Angela, I found my doughnut."

The sticky, smashed former maple bar was lodged perfectly between a pair of trays. When she lifted the tray she needed, it had also stuck to the tray underneath. After the smashed sugary remains dropped to the ground, Trisha was laughing so hard she couldn't get back on the phone to help her customer. The mystery of the missing maple bar was solved. Leave it to Bob.

## PSALM 62:6 NIV

He alone is my rock and my salvation; he is
my fortress, I will not be shaken.

Andrea made an appointment with a highly recommended nurse practitioner, Mickie Brennan, to confirm the pregnancy. She wanted to be sure to do everything right from the beginning to ensure a healthy baby. Sean kept telling her that if something's going to go wrong, then there's nothing you can do to prevent it. She knew that, but that didn't mean she would go out of her way to be unhealthy either. She was drinking water instead of colas; even cutting her daily thirty-two-ounce Dr. Pepper down to once a week at work. She was eating right and trying to keep her stress level under control.

Until about eight weeks along, Andrea herself wouldn't have any reason to suspect she was pregnant. Everything was great. Then the dreaded morning sickness showed its ugly face. She threw up every morning brushing her teeth. It got so bad sometimes she even skipped the tooth brushing. One morning at work, a deliveryman, Rusty, came in and told a tasteless joke that sent Andrea into hysterics. She had to run to the bathroom before she threw up in her garbage can. She threw up after lunch most days and felt nauseous the majority of the time. Although it was a disgusting feeling to be queasy all of the time, Andrea just figured it would pass at about three months along, as all of the books said it would. She had already read every pregnancy book she could get her hands on. Little did she know they would do her absolutely no good.

Andrea wanted a safer car to carry the baby in. She had been driving a Geo Metro hatchback for the last eight years. Not exactly the classy family vehicle she was looking for, but at a young age it was what she could afford and it had been a reliable car for her. She never had a problem with it. It was nice

*expect a miracle*  *19*

to have no car payment, and besides, the year before that, they had bought a new four-door Toyota pick-up for when they were ready to add to the family. On a Sunday afternoon, they went by the local Toyota dealership to check out some possible options for their new family rig. A few hours later, they came home with a Toyota Camry, a great four-door family car. The first thing Sean did to it was put new wheels on it. He couldn't be seen driving around in an old lady car, after all. To Andrea, it was driving in style, finally.

Both of them had good, steady jobs and they knew they were lucky. The unemployment rate in Oregon was one of the highest in the country and still rising. With dropping interest rates, they had been in the process of getting pre-approved for their first home. For some reason, after getting the approval, neither of them was as excited as they thought they would be. This was supposed to be a great thing and it scared them both. Their uneasiness was great enough that they both agreed to pass on the approval and wait a while. Hindsight would later tell them that was the best decision at the time.

It was fun to go out and begin buying the baby basics. They set up the crib. It was a pretty mahogany sleigh-style bed. Andrea couldn't help herself and put the bedding in to see what it would be like to lay the baby down in there. They bought things gradually, not all at once. They didn't even know whether they were having a boy or a girl yet. Their modest middle class accounts had plenty of money in them, and they were well prepared to purchase the things they would need and prepared for Andrea to be without her income during her maternity leave. Their life was perfect and getting better.

Sean went to her twelve-week check-up with her, and it was thrilling to hear the baby's heartbeat for the first time. Andrea had actually lost a pound, but that wasn't surprising, considering she couldn't keep any food down. Mickie checked around to listen for a possible second heartbeat, as she would always do, and ran across one in a different location, but it was the same rate as the one heard before, so she deduced that it was the same baby being heard. Mickie offered Andrea a prescription for the vomiting, but Andrea declined because she figured the morning sickness probably wouldn't last much longer. She continued trying everything people told her. From the obvious saltine crackers to drinking water, all of which came right back up. She found out later that water could actually upset your stomach even more!

About a week later, when she threw up her lunch at home for what seemed like the millionth time, she broke down crying and called the doctors office and asked them to call in the prescription for her. When she picked up the prescription, she saw the side effects on the bottle, which read, "Might cause upset stomach." She was sitting in the driver's seat in the grocery store parking lot and barely got the door open in time to vomit right beside her car. Not one of her shining moments. After taking the first pill, she threw up. It did help, though, gradually.

During the month of May, Sean began to get quite ill. He didn't have a primary care physician in Bend, although they had lived there for nearly five years. He was never sick and hadn't needed one. One evening after work, they went to the urgent care center one block from their home and the doctor requested some tests, but he didn't come up with a specific diagnosis. A couple of weeks later, Sean returned to the urgent care and it was determined he had a bronchial infection and he was put on an inhaler. By mid-June, he was so worn out and miserable, he returned yet again. The doctor had a whole battery of tests run and finally put his finger on the problem. Sean had developed Mono. He was told to stay home from work for

expect a miracle  *21*

at least a week, which wasn't a problem for Sean, because he barely had the energy to get out of bed.

While Sean was home with Mono, Andrea went to her sixteen-week check-up by herself. No reason for Sean to have to join her for this one. It was Wednesday, June 19. She still hadn't gained any weight, but she was huge. She was already wearing some maternity clothing. She and Mickie discussed possibly scheduling an ultrasound for the next month around week twenty. Mickie joked that she always needed a medical reason to request an ultrasound, so she wrote down that Andrea measured a "little big." The exam continued and Andrea's belly was measured. She was told that she was, in fact, bigger than expected. All Andrea said was, "I thought so. I've already started to wear some maternity clothes."

Mickie told her at that gestation her belly should measure about sixteen centimeters, around one centimeter per week. Well, Andrea measured twenty-one centimeters! Mickie listened for a heartbeat and found it right away. She moved around Andrea's belly to listen for more and heard what sounded a little different. She listened for what seemed to Andrea to be quite a while, but never led Andrea to believe she was concerned. She told her it could be twins or maybe just an enlarged placenta. She emphasized a need to get in for an ultrasound soon. They discussed how soon Andrea would like to have it done. Andrea figured that Fridays were usually the easiest days to leave work early and said to try for that Friday. Mickie told her she called the hospital and they could get her in on Thursday, the very next morning, at 11:00 AM

Andrea said, "Sure."

Mickie told her she was relieved that Andrea had chosen not to wait until Friday. It would make for a long wait.

Andrea soon found out that even waiting until eleven o'clock the next morning seemed torturous. She told the girls at work they were waiting until eleven, and they got into discussions of what it could be. Of course, everyone thought it could be twins, although neither Andrea nor Sean had reason to believe that twins ran in their families. The girls began to joke about all kinds of possibilities. Trisha hoped it was twins. Elizabeth said that just wouldn't cut it. It would have to be triplets so they could each have one. Andrea said her fear was that she had a baby with a giant head. Trisha followed with, "No, it's an octopus baby!"

"Yeah, okay. It's probably nothing at all, so stop scaring me," Andrea said.

Little did anyone realize they would all be right in their own strange way.

Before the appointment, Andrea went by the house and picked up a very worn out Sean and drove to the hospital where they would have the ultrasound. It was an exciting time for two first-time parents. They had decided that if it was visible, they would find out the sex of the baby. Mimi was their sonographer and was a friendly, thin young lady with long blonde hair. She asked the couple if they were told anything. Andrea told her they thought it was possibly twins or an enlarged placenta.

Mimi said, "Okay," and began the ultrasound. Andrea's belly was completely exposed with hand towels tucked into her clothes to prevent the gel from staining them. Mimi covered Andrea with warm, sticky gel. She began to use the hand piece to spread the gel and get a quick overview of the uterus. She immediately said, "Yep, there's two."

Andrea looked at Sean and smiled, but they quickly turned back to the screen to watch their babies. After scanning the area for a few more minutes in silence, Mimi said with uneasy breath, "Well, I see three heads, but only two bodies."

Andrea's eyes couldn't leave the screen, but her left hand

expect a miracle *23*

reached out to the side where Sean sat in shock and found a place tucked in his much larger hand.

There's an expression used every day and it's taken for granted. People say their "mind went blank." Sean and Andrea discovered what it actually meant to have your mind go blank. The feeling of shock didn't hit immediately. They both stared at the monitor without a thought or rationalization of what was going on. As Mimi continued to scan over the area and get a feel for what she was looking at, even she was unsure of the consequences of this pregnancy. She had never personally seen conjoined twins before, let alone with a triplet involved also, and tried to proceed as she thought best. She asked the couple if they wanted her to explain what she saw as she went along. They said yes. She started with the single baby, labeled "baby A," and that was straight forward. It was strange to feel excited at these first images of their babies, but the uneasiness of the unknown was overwhelming.

As Mimi measured arms, legs, and general body length, she asked them if they wanted to know the sex. They both said that they had already decided to learn the sex if possible and agreed it couldn't hurt now. She positioned the monitor again to gain a better view, and Sean and Andrea could both see it was a boy. After getting all of the images and measurements that were standard for a single baby, Mimi moved on to the conjoined twins. She explained their shared anatomy as best she could while she tried to make sense of it. Labeling one side "baby B" and the other "baby C," she began with the measurements that could be taken separately. These babies were also boys. They shared almost their entire body, with two heads, at least one arm on each side of the shoulders, and possibly a third limb behind and between the heads. There were two spines going down into a shared torso, three hip bones, and only two legs. As for internal organs, the babies were so small that it was hard to read. They appeared to have two stomachs, at least two, maybe three kidneys, and two partially joined hearts. Watching those two babies move and wiggle was awe-inspiring. The experience of wondering how this could happen to a young, healthy couple who tried to do everything right was mind-boggling.

### EPHESIANS 1:11 NIV

In him we were also chosen, having been predestined according to the plan of him who works out everything in conformity with the purpose of his will.

After Mimi took all of the appropriate measurements, she handed Andrea a towel to wipe off some of the gel but told her to stay put because they might need to look at the babies a little bit more. Before walking out, she also handed her a box of tissues and a few pictures she had printed out of the babies. Sean and Andrea didn't know what to say to each other once they were alone. Andrea looked at the clock. It was one o'clock, the time she ordered lenses every day. She said, "I hope Trisha orders lenses for me."

Mimi returned about ten minutes later with the head of radiology, who sat down to take a look for himself. By the end of the three-hour long ultrasound, Andrea was tired of lying on the table and being covered with gel. Sean was mentally exhausted from taking it all in. They were told that Andrea's nurse midwife's office had been called, and they were to meet her and another doctor at that office at three o'clock that afternoon to discuss the findings. So they went home to wait.

At home, Sean lay down on the living room floor with a comforter and Andrea just sat on the floor with her knees up and her back against the couch. She knew the people at work would be pacing the floor to know what was taking so long.

expect a miracle *25*

When she called, Trisha answered the phone and yelled, "Where have you been?"

Andrea proceeded to tell her they had one sac with a healthy baby boy in it and another sac with Siamese twins. Trisha didn't know what to say. Andrea told her she would talk to her later since they had to meet with her doctors in a little while.

Trisha and Elizabeth went into John's office and shut the door. They were all stunned by the new information, feeling absolutely horrified by the comments they were making before the appointment. Each of them had tears in their eyes and it was agreed, for the time being, it was not to be discussed with anyone outside of that room.

A little while later, the newest employee, Dave, who had only been hired about two weeks prior as a data entry person asked, "How did the appointment go?"

Elizabeth just responded with, "I think things have taken a turn for the worse."

As the afternoon went on and they continued with their duties, the mood was so solemn that John thought he would lighten the air. He placed a remote control fart machine in the recycle bin that was located between the copy machine and Trisha's desk. While Elizabeth was making copies, John used the remote from around the corner in his office. Neither girl said anything, so John did it again. Elizabeth was afraid Trisha would think it was she, and they both started to look for where it was coming from. At that moment, John could contain himself no longer and busted out laughing from his office. The rest of the day went a little bit better for the three of them.

At three o'clock, the couple went to the doctor's office and were escorted right in without a wait. They were met by Mickie Brennan and Dr. Mary Jane Davis. Mickie told them the situation had gone beyond her area of expertise as a certified nurse

26  andrea merkord

midwife, but she would still be available to help if they needed anything. She introduced them to Dr. Davis, who explained their situation in a frank and straightforward manner, which was how they liked being spoken to. She discussed the anatomy of the twins, which they had already been made aware of during the ultrasound. They were made aware of an additional problem though.

The babies suffered from a condition called Twin to Twin Transfusion Syndrome. This occurs in identical twin settings, or higher sets of multiples, when the babies share a placenta. Amongst all of the vessels and arteries in the placenta, some of them become shared during a very early growth period. In some rare cases, there is an uneven amount of blood sharing between the babies. This causes life-threatening conditions, including anemia and heart failure.

Dr. Davis told them she had been in contact with Dr. Elaine Di Federico, a perinatologist in Portland, all afternoon and they were trying to schedule a time to get them in as soon as possible. They were given the number to the office in Portland and the name of Kevin, the person they were to contact at nine o'clock the next morning to see if they had an appointment yet. They went home with more news to ponder.

Sean called his mom and tried to explain what was found to the best of his ability.

She told him, "Thomas is a strong name and he'll be a strong boy."

Thomas was one of a few names they had been considering for their baby if they had a boy. From that moment on, his name was definitely Thomas. Carol had the duty to call other family members and let them know the news.

Andrea called her sister Amber and told her also. After a short discussion about what they would do, it was up to Amber to call the rest of their family and share the news. After Amber

expect a miracle    27

had called their dad at home after work, he went out to his dad's fifth wheel. Roger and Bobbie were up in Oregon visiting the family during the summer and always parked their fifth wheel at Steve and Mary's house just outside of the pool area where they could "plug in." Steve asked Bobbie to come out to the shop so they could talk. He didn't want his dad to see him cry. After telling her what he could, he just hugged her as he wept. He told Mary when she returned home from work that night. That was the beginning of long cycles of telephone calls that would be made from family member to family member as new information was received. It was a great relief to Sean and Andrea, because to repeat the story was much too difficult.

A little bit after five that night, they heard a knock on the door. It was Trisha. She hugged Andrea as soon as she opened the door. Trisha joined them on the living room floor, and it was a pretty solemn sight. Sean's eyes were filled with tears and Trisha leaned over to give him a big hug. As was Trisha's nature, she couldn't help but bring a little humor into their lives. They got into inappropriate conversations about how you would raise conjoined twins and what life would be like with them. It was a moment between just the three of them, because even though the laughter was what they desperately needed, the jokes would most likely not be appreciated by any others outside of the group. It was a good escape for a few short minutes though. When their thoughts returned to the reality of it all, it was strange to ponder what kind of life conjoined twins would be faced with. What if they did survive? That thought was almost scarier than the thought of them not making it. What would their quality of life be? Would Sean and Andrea have the means to care for them if they were in need of full time medical care? Could they play with other children, or even their brother? Would Thomas be brushed aside because the twins required all of the attention?

Andrea got on-line later that night to look up internet sites about conjoined twins. The statistics were amazing. There is a 1 in 200,000 chance of having conjoined twins. Most conjoined twins are female. Fifty percent of all conjoined twins die in-utero. Of the ones that do survive until birth, thirty-five percent of those will die within twenty-four hours. When combined with the 1 in 8,100 chance of having naturally conceived triplets, not to mention identical triplets, complicated with the rare chances of having Twin-Twin Transfusion Syndrome, the odds of this pregnancy even taking place were off the charts, and it became much rarer as time went on.[1]

Elizabeth left work with the daunting task of sharing the frightening information with Leah. Leah was her eleven-year-old daughter and old enough to understand the dreadfulness of the news, but still young enough to be terrified by what she was hearing.

They sat down on the couch and Lizzy said, "I need you to sit with me for a minute."

Leah listened as Elizabeth went through the day's findings. They were both crushed by the news that this was happening to their friend.

Leah looked up and said to her mom, "Andrea is very special to be chosen to carry those babies."

She also got on the internet that same night and began to look up the sites on conjoined twins. Being a very intelligent young girl, she wanted to make sure she really understood what was going on.

Friday morning, Sean and Andrea woke up early. Neither of them really slept. Andrea sat on the bed, phone and organizer in her lap, next to where Sean was still lying. It was only six o'clock and she wasn't supposed to call the doctor's office in Portland until nine o'clock. Time seemed to be in slow motion. Luckily, the phone rang at eight-forty and it was Kevin from

expect a miracle   *29*

Portland. The schedule was very full and they had to do some shuffling just to get them in. They had an appointment scheduled for first thing Monday morning. First, they would go to the diagnostic center of Emanuel Hospital to have an ultrasound and then continue upstairs to the office to consult with the doctor. They were to be there at eight o'clock. Andrea got directions to the hospital and all of the phone numbers she might need. Now, all they could do was wait out the long weekend that inevitably had to come before Monday.

Sean's parents were planning on driving up to Washington to spend the weekend with their oldest daughter, Karla, and her family to celebrate granddaughter Jordyn's fifth birthday. Sean and Andrea decided it would be a great way to pass the time, and they would be closer to Portland when Monday came around. They packed, stopped by Andrea's work to drop off a house key for Trisha, who was happy to feed their cat for them and get the mail, and drove to Albany (of course, Andrea threw up on the side of the road not long into their drive) and then rode up I-5 with Tony and Carol (Andrea threw up in the car about halfway through that drive all over her pillowcase). It was a lot of driving for one day.

Saturday was Jordyn's birthday party and there were many of her friends there to join in. Her younger brother, Taylor, hung out as well. They had rented a play gym called a "Jumpy-Jump" that was a large blown-up cage the children went into and bounced around in. Sean, Andrea, Karla, and her husband, Martin, even got in.

During lunch, one of Karla's friends strolled up with a set of twin girls in a stroller. They ended up talking about the fact that Andrea had triplets and the lady gave her all kinds of advice on how to get deals on multiple cribs, clothes, and various baby needs. After a few minutes, Andrea made a quiet exit back into the house and sat alone wondering what would happen to her three babies. Would she even get the chance to worry about all of that?

They already had one crib set up. Would they get to use it at all? Andrea was surprised at a feeling of jealousy she had when seeing the attention the other mother got about her twin girls. She wondered why it couldn't have just been twins. Why did it get so screwed up? Actually, *how* did it get so screwed up? They didn't have any of the answers that she desperately needed. All they could think about on Sunday was the upcoming appointment on Monday. Andrea slept most of the day. Sunday night they drove back to Albany to stay at Tony and Carol's house.

### DEUTERONOMY 31:8 NIV

The Lord himself goes before you and will be with you; he will never leave you nor forsake you. Do not be afraid; do not be discouraged.

Monday morning, on the one hour drive to Portland, they put in a peaceful Christian CD they listened to often. Andrea rested her head on Sean's shoulder and cried. The directions to the hospital were surprisingly easy and they got there in plenty of time. They went directly to the diagnostic center and checked in. After the usual paperwork that would become excruciatingly redundant over the next year, they returned to the waiting room and had a seat.

It occurred to Andrea that no person in the room knew why they were there. They would have no idea these two young people were going through the most difficult time of their lives, faced with the horrifying and grim future that would paralyze the mind of any person who tried to ponder it for any extended period of time. To the casual passerby, they were just a happy couple expecting a baby and were there for an ultrasound. From that point on, Andrea looked at other people

expect a miracle *31*

through different eyes. They could be having the best or the worst day of their lives. What people say or how they treat others can and does have a direct impact on them. Whether it's a bad look or a gesture or a rude comment made under the breath, but purposely loud enough to be heard, it can crush an already breaking heart. A smile can go miles.

She tried to remember to offer more smiles to strangers, and even more importantly, to family, co-workers, and friends. Having a face-to-face battle with pain and heartache is one of the best ways to become a more empathetic person. Instead of judging someone for their actions, maybe they would be better helped with support.

They were soon called into the sonogram room. This hospital was different, and the technician didn't discuss the scan as she went along. It was another two-and-a-half-hour ultrasound followed by the head of the department coming in to look at it further. They found out more specific information about the anatomy of the twins. There was, indeed, a limb between the heads. Inside this one little arm were all of the bones for two complete arms. At the end were two tiny, but perfectly formed hands. Andrea had a difficult time lying on her back for that long. The weight of her uterus was too much. They periodically allowed her to shift or even lean to one side to accommodate her comfort. Sean could see the different measurements being taken. They watched as they measured the amount of fluid surrounding the babies.

Sean and Andrea were sent upstairs to meet with the perinatologist, a gynecologist who specializes in complicated pregnancies. They were escorted into a small exam room, but after a short time, the nurse told them it would be a while and they should go downstairs to get some lunch. If they only knew, as they found their way to the cafeteria, they would soon know their way up and down many of the halls of this hospital. After

32   andrea merkord

lunch, the couple was very tired and still had a meeting with the doctor to look forward to. While they waited, Andrea read all of the papers the nurses had given her about multiple pregnancies and Twin-Twin Transfusion Syndrome.

Some of the information they received was from The Twin To Twin Transfusion Syndrome Foundation. It explained their situation in six pages of extensive clinical details:

## WHAT IS TWIN TO TWIN TRANSFUSION SYNDROME?

- Twin to twin transfusion syndrome (TTTS) is a random disease of the placenta.
- It affects identical twins during pregnancy with a monochorionic (MC) placenta, or shared placenta.
- It is occurring when blood passes disproportionately from one baby to the other through connecting blood vessels within their shared placenta.
- Identical twins usually share blood flow when they share a monochorionic placenta, but approximately 15% of the time, the sharing of blood is so unequal that the one baby gets too much blood flow, and the other too little.
- The recipient twin is the baby that gets too much blood. The recipient becomes larger in size because of the excessive amounts of blood. The recipient's blood becomes very thick like syrup and the baby's heart has to pump much harder to get the blood through his system. The baby's cardiovascular system may become so overloaded that heart failure begins.
- The donor baby is the one that gets too little blood. The donor may become very anemic due

expect a miracle   33

to the lower volume of blood. The donor at birth often does better than the recipient, because he is not as tired.

• Twin to twin transfusion syndrome is predetermined to happen soon after conception when the umbilical cords randomly attach to the placenta and the blood vessels become shared. It is just unknown at what gestation week in the pregnancy that these connections will be triggered to cause problems.

• Chronic twin to twin transfusion syndrome typically presents itself in the mid-second trimester. The earlier the diagnosis (16–26 weeks) the more serious the condition simply because the babies cannot be delivered and have a longer time to be affected by the disease. Left without treatment, one or more babies may not survive. With treatment, their odds of survival drastically improve. By destroying the abnormal placental blood vessels that connect the twins, laser surgery is the only method which can halt or limit the effects of the twin to twin transfusion syndrome on the babies. Being diagnosed prior to twenty-six weeks is more serious. With all the excessive amniotic fluid the mother is at increased risk for pre-term labor so this needs to be addressed and treatments need to be pursued and implemented immediately. Some women are measuring full-term and/or may show heart failure already in the babies. Sadly, some MC twins may have shares of the common placenta that are unable to sustain their lives in the womb to a point where they can survive if delivered. When this twin passes away, the other twin is at risk for death or birth defects because of the connecting vessels. The only therapy that can remove these risks to the other twin is laser surgery because it can "disconnect" the MC twins.[2]

It was two hours before the doctor came in. Dr. Difederico was a thin, middle-aged woman with very short graying hair. She had a calm and friendly demeanor with a soft smile on her face. She went over their situation with them and explained the complications being caused by the Twin-Twin Transfusion Syndrome. In Andrea's case, the twins were labeled as "the donor" and the single boy was labeled as "the recipient." The donor babies were pushing extra amounts of blood over to the other baby, causing themselves to be dehydrated and extremely anemic. Their sac had almost no fluid in it. They had very little room to move freely. In that case, they are often referred to as the "stuck" twin. It's as if they were wrapped in plastic wrap. The recipient baby was receiving the extra amounts of blood and his efforts to keep up with it could cause him to have heart failure because of the pressure caused by the excessive amounts of fluid in his sac.

Dr. Di Federico laid out their limited options.

1) They could terminate the pregnancy. When this option was brought up, Andrea just started to cry and said they had just gotten finished watching three babies moving around, alive and kicking. Sean and Andrea didn't want to do that.

2) They could have fluid reductions. They would have to come back to Portland every couple of weeks to have fluid taken out of the sac of the

expect a miracle  35

single baby. The procedure is basically a glorified amniocentesis, when they draw out a small amount of amniotic fluid to run tests. Instead, they just remove large amounts of fluid each time. Unfortunately, this procedure runs the risk of pre-term labor each time it's done and doesn't solve the bigger problem. It treats the symptom but is not a cure. This still didn't answer the question of if the twins were to die in-utero, what would happen to the other baby? He would soon follow due to the sharing of blood.

3) They could check into having surgery performed in San Francisco by doctors who have been doing risky fetal surgeries on pregnant women for twenty years. These surgeries were only performed at a few hospitals in the country. There was no guarantee that Sean and Andrea would even be a candidate for a surgery, but the doctor could call and talk to them if they wanted her to.

The doctor briefly mentioned that there was a hospital in Philadelphia with doctors who have separated Siamese twins before. It probably wouldn't be an option considering the shared anatomy of their twins, however. Faced with the additional complications, they probably would never get the chance to find out anyway.

Unhappy with the choices, Andrea asked, "What if we do nothing?"

Dr. Di Federico said, "That is always an option. There is a ninety to one hundred percent chance that they would all die."

Faced with those odds, Sean and Andrea told her to go

ahead and contact the doctors in San Francisco. She had their number and said she would have Dr. Sandberg, a former associate of hers, give them a call the next day.

# THE DARK SIDE OF JOY

**ISAIAH 43:2 NIV**
When you pass through the waters, I will be with you;
and when you pass through the rivers, they will not
sweep over you. When you walk through the fire, you will
not be burned; the flames will not set you ablaze.

*A*fter a long day in Portland, Sean and Andrea drove back to Albany to Sean's parents' house. Neither of them felt up to a long drive back to Bend, so they decided to stay the night in Albany again. On Tuesday, they checked their messages all day, waiting for a call from the doctor in San Francisco. Sean also had Wednesday off of work already and asked Andrea if she wouldn't mind staying another night at his parents' house. She called work to check with them and John said they could really use her. She didn't want to be a burden to her coworkers and told Sean they really needed to head home. Sean became upset and sad and told her that with everything running through his mind, this was the place he could come to to feel safe and secure, the place he had spent eighteen years of his life. She didn't want to play the bad guy, and called John again, crying, and said they really needed an extra day away. John said that it was fine.

Sean called to check their messages again in the early afternoon, and there was finally a message from Dr. Sandberg. Andrea returned his call and left messages at both of the numbers she was given, telling him they would be at a different number until tomorrow. They were sitting in the grass in the backyard of Tony and Carol's home with the cell phone while they kept Andrea's day-timer handy with all of the numbers they needed at their fingertips. They didn't hear from him again that night. Waiting for the phone to ring was exhausting. They just visited while they tried to pass the time.

When they returned home on Wednesday, they had already missed another call from the doctor. There was also a message from Carol, who he had called also, in which she stated the doctor would call them back at home at five-thirty. They felt horrible playing phone tag with a doctor who they knew must be a very busy man. Hanna, their eight-year-old Persian cat, was excited to see them after being away for five days. Andrea was usually good about Hanna's care and brushed her long hair regularly. Hanna would put up with it for a while and would get up with an attitude when she decided she had had enough, taunting with her tail as she slinked away.

Sean went to pick up some dinner at Taco Bell, while Andrea waited for the phone call. They were determined not to miss it this time. She was sitting on the ground in front of the cocktail table, the phone at arm's reach, and a pen and pad of paper handy to make notes. Dr. Sandberg called at ten minutes after six. When the phone rang, Andrea's heart nearly leaped out of her chest. She had written down a list of questions they had and was very anxious to talk to him. He informed her there were two possible procedures they could do, but they wouldn't know which one would be best for them until they got to San Francisco. She was concerned about recovery time, and he explained with one procedure, it would be one or two days in the hospital with a week of rest. With the other procedure, it could be many days in the hospital. Andrea was hoping for the shortest stay possible and a quick return to work. He told her they needed to come as soon as possible. They were to call Jody at his office in the morning to arrange for appoint-

expect a miracle   *39*

ments, and travel, and accommodations. Andrea made sure to do all of their laundry so they would be ready to pack again whenever necessary.

Thursday started out like any other day. They both went to work and Andrea waited until eight-thirty to go into John's office and call Jody in San Francisco. Jody said she would arrange for an ultrasound Friday, and they needed to get down there that night. Andrea had to fax all of her insurance information to the hospital to get pre-approval. Jody faxed back to her a list of lodging in the immediate area of the hospital. Andrea called Sean and asked him to arrange for airfare that afternoon and she would handle hotels. After briefly perusing the list, Andrea settled on a bed and breakfast that was directly across the street from the hospital and only ninety-nine dollars a night.

Sean called a travel agent they had used before, Nancy, but the prices she quoted were too much, some were four hundred dollars per person. Sean chose to go another avenue and got online. He found round trip tickets for them for only $119 per person! The down side was that the flight left out of Portland at five PM that afternoon. Sean called Andrea at work at ten forty-five and told her she had to leave *"right now!"*

Andrea barely said good-byes and rushed home. Luckily, she only worked ten minutes from home. Sean was even closer. They were packed and leaving the house by eleven fifteen.

On the way out of town, they stopped to get food and, of course, Andrea threw up just past Sisters, a small tourist town just west of Bend. They stopped by a bank on the way and took out a thousand dollars. Better to be prepared for any circumstance. They would use that money to pay for everything. Sean had arranged for them to drive to Albany first to meet Tony. Since they didn't know what day they would be returning, this gave them a place to leave their car. They met at Home Depot right next to the freeway at two fifteen. Later that evening, Tony and Carol would come back and pick up the car and take it home with them. The drive to the Portland airport from Albany usually took about an hour and a half. That would give them enough time for the check in, which had become quite an ordeal since the September 11 attacks the previous year. About fifteen minutes up interstate 5, just south of Salem, they came upon a traffic jam that had nearly reached a halt. Andrea kept looking at a delivery truck that advertised Icees, which sounded really good right then. Their hearts sank as they sat there for forty minutes before moving again.

They arrived at the airport at five minutes after four. Tony offered his cell phone to them to use while they were away because he had unlimited minutes during week nights and weekends. Since they had no time, their good-bye was a quick one. Luckily, they had electronic tickets, so that sped up the process as well. Before boarding the plane, they heard the announcement that there would be random bag checks during boarding and they should quietly step aside if asked to do so. Sean watched as a Muslim family was pulled aside to have their carry-on bags checked and wondered exactly how "random" it really was.

The flight to San Francisco was uneventful, and they arrived at six forty-five. It was already sunset as they took a cab from the airport to their hotel. Neither of them had much experience with taxi cabs. They were both raised in much smaller cities than this one. This driver went so fast in and out of lanes and up and down the hilly streets of San Francisco, Andrea fought to keep from vomiting. He wasn't quite sure where the bed and breakfast was once they reached the hospital but found the street in just a couple of minutes. Sean was blown away when the cab fare was forty dollars.

They were left standing on the sidewalk of a dark street

that looked like a small neighborhood of apartments. They walked up the steps to the office, which was closed for the day. To their left was a small black mailbox with two sets of papers in it. They pulled out the set with their last name on it and inside were a key and directions to their room. At first, they couldn't find the right building, but after a few minutes, they made their way back toward the office and ran across it. They had to use a key to open the main door and walked up the stairs directly in front of them. They were in the room to the right of the top of the stairs, right next to the bathroom. When they opened the door and turned on the light, Sean's face turned sour. Neither of them had ever stayed in a bed and breakfast before, but this place was a dive. The room was so small there was barely enough room for the bed. Paint was chipping off the walls and the closet door looked like it was about to fall off the hinges. On one end of the tattered dresser was an ancient television set with black rabbit ears on top of it. They both shook their heads in disappointment.

Next door, the bathroom wasn't any better. They weren't used to sharing a bathroom with other guests. There was a tiny room with a lone toilet and a rickety ol' window overhead behind that. Next to that was a room with the shower and a sink. The shower was like the one in the movie *Psycho*, with a curtain that wrapped around it. Andrea refused to shower in there alone and they bathed together that night.

Amongst the papers that were left for them at the office was a fax from Jody at the hospital. It informed them of their eight AM ultrasound the following morning. There were also directions to that area of campus and a shuttle schedule. Andrea was afraid they would miss the shuttle since the clock in their room wasn't digital and the alarm didn't work. Not to worry though, who could sleep anyway?

Sean scanned through the whopping three channels the TV

had and the only thing that was on was news. They were both shocked to discover the gay pride parade was that weekend. They weren't used being in such a liberal environment. There was also going to be an increase in the toll fare for the Golden Gate Bridge. Good to know.

They were both starving and pulled out the phone book to order in a pizza or something. Trying various names in the phone book, they had to find one that delivered to the area, and they had no idea what area of town it was. They settled on a pizza parlor and ordered pepperoni and some Root Beer. The delivery guy even got lost locating them, but eventually found the bed and breakfast. Sean had to go downstairs to let him in. Andrea was waiting cross-legged on the bed ready to chow down. When they were settled and finally ripped into the pizza, they were totally let down again. It was practically flavorless, and they basically ate it just to get some food in their bellies. The only good thing about that day was the Root Beer. They both figured they might be admitted to the hospital the next day, so at least they only had to stay in that room one night. The best thing they could do was to try to get some rest.

## NAHUM 1:7 NIV

The Lord is good, a refuge in times of trouble.
He cares for those who trust in him.

Early Friday morning, they were up and ready to go find a shuttle to their appointment. They asked one shuttle driver, who was stopped, where the Mount Zion location was, and he told them which shuttle to get on. That was very helpful, because it was stressful to be on a time schedule but have no idea where they were going or how long it would take to get there.

Once they were on the right shuttle, they passed by a

expect a miracle   43

park with a man in a grassy area doing some type of oriental exercises. Not a sight they were used to in their hometown. They arrived at the Mount Zion campus in plenty of time and asked at the front desk where to go from there. Upstairs, they were the first to arrive. It was about a quarter 'til eight and the office wasn't open yet. Sean sat down at the end of the hall on the ground beneath a window. Andrea found a bathroom just across from the office door and barely made it there before she threw up heavily. Her eyes were watering, and she wondered how bad this whole ordeal would get. As she looked around the small rectangular bathroom, she was disturbed; it was a medical center and it was in total disrepair. The walls had chipping paint and had some spaces and cracks in the corners. She began to realize that maybe it was an older part of the city of San Francisco.

Once they were let into the office, they sat in the waiting area together rather nervously. There was an Asian lady who arrived for her appointment, and when asked by the woman at the desk to repeat her name, Sean and Andrea both looked at each other and at the same moment whispered, "The heck you say."

They laughed, not at the name itself, but at the fact that they had said the words at precisely the same moment. It felt good to laugh.

Andrea heard a woman come from the back of the office asking for the chart for "the triplets." Andrea knew she must be referring to them. The first two hours of the ultrasound were done by a lady who didn't talk very much about what she was seeing. Andrea spent the entire time checking out the elaborately painted ceiling. It was eye catching and looked like a tide pool or underwater view. She also watched the monitor quite a bit, even though they were very quickly getting used to the awe-inspiring sights on the screen. That was followed by another gentleman coming in to get some more pictures. Andrea was getting so uncomfortable lying on her back, she kept shifting her weight. She felt like a child who couldn't hold still. She was trying very hard not to bother the technician so he could do his job. She was feeling sick to her stomach and told Sean to grab the garbage can. Rolling over the edge of the table, she threw up into the can. The man gave her a towel to wipe her mouth with and left the room to give her minute to sit up. She was so embarrassed and felt bad for doing that in front of him.

After the ultrasound, they got back on the shuttle and returned to the main hospital building to meet with Dr. Sandberg. It was Moffitt-Long hospital. One side was Moffitt hospital, and the other was Long hospital. Andrea was lost in a place that large, so it didn't matter to her what the name was. They were first taken to a small exam room where Andrea was told to put on a gown. She was confused as to why, and the nurse said she would be right back. The nurse came back and apologized; they didn't need an exam, so she took them back to the main desk of the labor and delivery ward. It was a long counter with hustling nurses and staffing working busily. They were told to go downstairs to the cafeteria to get something to eat and return at eleven thirty.

The cafeteria was large with areas for pizza, salad bar, and a variety of other choices. It was about three times the size of the cafeteria at Emanuel Hospital in Portland. At eleven thirty, they returned to the fifteenth floor and were escorted to a large labor room to wait for the doctor. For three long hours the couple took turns lying down on the small couch to snooze and spent some time looking out the window at the bay. Finally, at two thirty, Dr. Sandberg came into the room and introduced himself. He was a tall middle-aged man with a medium build, round belly that you could see through his blue scrubs, and short dark hair with grey tips. He discussed the two possible procedures with them and drew quaint diagrams to help them better understand what he was saying.

In either procedure, the incisions on Andrea's belly and uterus would be extremely small. With the first option, they would go in and basically cauterize the cord to the twins. This would cut off their blood supply, which would stop the sharing of blood between them and the third baby, Thomas, but would also cause their demise. With the second option, they would actually search out the various connecting vessels and arteries and cut each one individually. This procedure was much more risky, time consuming, and would cause a longer hospital stay as well. Dr. Sandberg needed to go downstairs to look at their ultrasound pictures and then he would return.

Sean re-booked their room at the bed and breakfast for one more night. He needed to run across the street to get their bags back in their room before the office closed at five. They were holding their bags in the office for them until they were finished. Andrea waited in the labor room upstairs just in case the doctor came back before they had returned from their room across the street. While Sean was still gone, Dr. Sandberg did come back and told her she needed to go downstairs with him to have an amnio reduction.

At three forty-five, Sean and Andrea went down to the third floor and easily found the doctor. He was in an ultrasound room getting ready to take out some of Andrea's excess fluid. They were told the low risks of the procedure, which included premature rupture of membranes and miscarriage at that early stage. Andrea was afraid of needles and was scared out of her mind but tried not to let it show to the doctor and his two students, who were there to help and learn. One student shook the couple's hands and introduced himself before helping Dr.

Sandberg. The other student stood off to the side and stayed out of the way.

Dr. Sandberg started out by using the ultrasound to locate the best place to go in with the needle. He marked it on her belly and gave her a local anesthetic to numb the skin before inserting the much larger needle. Andrea never looked at the syringe but was so nervous that she had a couple of tears that escaped her eyes no matter how hard she tried to stop them. She watched Sean, who was watching the needle wide-eyed. They had sucked out 1350 milliliters of fluid before they were finished. Sean saw one and a half glass jars of amniotic fluid out of Thomas's sac sitting on the counter. It looked like urine.

Dr. Sandberg explained it might allow more fluid to build in the sac of the twins, making the operation easier to do. It would also release pressure off of Thomas. They would be doing the first procedure discussed. It was determined by the staff to be the safer option for everyone involved. Then came the bad news. They would not be having surgery until Tuesday! They needed to be at the hospital Saturday morning for a follow up ultrasound to check the fluid. The soonest they would be able to leave San Francisco would be the following Thursday.

They had a lot to think about and decided to eat dinner at the cafeteria for convenience sake before returning to their room across the street. Their return ticket home was for that Saturday. That was the date Sean booked it for on-line, because it gave him the cheapest tickets down from Oregon. Because it was a discounted ticket, they were not able to change their tickets home to a later date. They discussed the possibility of going home after the ultrasound the next morning and flying back for surgery on Tuesday or booking a hotel for the next three nights. After comparing the expense factor, neither option was more financially beneficial than the other. They eventually opted to stay for the simple reason that traveling

expect a miracle   47

back and forth would just add more stress to an already uptight couple. Sean called and cancelled their flight home.

### ROMANS 8:28 NIV

And we know that in all things God works for the good of those who love him, who have been called according to his purpose.

Saturday morning, Sean and Andrea decided to take advantage of the complimentary breakfast provided at the bed and breakfast. It was just downstairs from them. They sat at a quaint table in a small room with a group of hoity-toity people who were on vacation. The room was overflowing with gaudy trinkets, like a little antique shop. Sean was relieved to be checking out, even though they had no idea where they would be staying that night.

Andrea called her boss, Scott, in Boise, Idaho, at home to update him about their unplanned extended stay in San Francisco. He was gone, but his wife, Bonnie, answered the phone. Andrea didn't know her well, but she was kind and interested in their well-being. They had a great conversation, and it was uplifting to Andrea to talk to another Christian about their circumstances.

At the follow-up ultrasound, it appeared the fluid reduction had gone well and the twins might even have had more fluid around them already. The personnel in the department gave them a phone book and a desk to use so they could find accommodations for the next three nights. They opted for a Courtyard Marriott that was located in South San Francisco. Not close to the hospital, but a relief to stay at a place of which they knew the name. Sean decided it would be good for them to feel some relaxation during this time and booked a king suite with a Jacuzzi tub in the corner of their room, a poolroom, spa, and on-site restaurant and laundry service. They thanked the people on the third floor for all of their help and went to call a cab downstairs.

The cab driver who picked them up was an older lady with one long earring in the shape of a skeleton. After talking with her for only a couple of minutes, they both felt comfortable with her, despite the earring. She asked why they were in San Francisco, and they gave her a brief explanation. She was so blown away by their story; she gave them a card with her cell phone number on it and told them to call her on Tuesday if they needed a ride back to the hospital. They were so appreciative and thanked her for the ride.

As soon as they were checked into their room, they both felt a huge load off. It was a nice room and more like what they were accustomed to. It felt more like home. The first thing Sean did was get into the Jacuzzi. They weren't quite sure what they were going to do about dinner. When they stepped outside to view their surroundings, they realized they were staying in a new development and there was absolutely nothing within walking distance. They went down to the front desk, and the lady there was very helpful and gave them menus for ordering in. She also listed a couple of fast food restaurants that were fairly close and offered to have the hotel shuttle drive them down to Wendy's. They took her up on that offer and picked up some burgers and drinks. Once they were settled in for the night, they looked at the list of movie rentals available on the TV and decided to rent *The Lord of the Rings*. Sean got into the Jacuzzi again and Andrea realized she didn't have anything to wear in the Jacuzzi herself. It wasn't like they had packed for a vacation. She decided since they were in the privacy of their own room that she would go in it in her birthday suit. She made sure the water wasn't too hot, considering her delicate condition.

Sunday was as uneventful a day as they had had in a short

expect a miracle   49

while. They went down to the hotel restaurant to have the breakfast buffet, which turned out to be very good. They had a large variety to choose from. After breakfast, they decided to wash their clothes since they hadn't packed enough to stay for that long. While the laundry was going, Sean spent some time in the pool. There wasn't any way for Andrea to go in, so she sat on the side and stuck her feet in the water while talking to Sean.

Andrea said, "I don't think it's really fair that you get to be all relaxed in the pool when I'm the one who has to have surgery. I'm the one carrying our babies and I can't even relax!"

Sean laughed at her sitting on the side and gloated while he swam away with a big grin on his face.

After an exciting morning of laundry, they went to the lobby and picked up cold sandwiches for lunch. They couldn't do any sort of sightseeing for two reasons. One, they couldn't waste the money, and they quickly realized how much taxi cabs cost. Two, Andrea was supposed to be taking it easy after the amniotic fluid reduction they had on Friday afternoon. They spent the day watching a lot of TV. It was definitely more relaxing than the tiny bed and breakfast. Relaxation was their goal in staying at that hotel, even though it was much farther from the hospital.

They both spent a large amount of time on the phone with family members, giving the latest updates on the situation. Andrea described to Amber what the fluid reduction was like, and pregnant April was thankful she didn't have to go through it. Sean called his parents and talked for a while about what the plans were as of then. They had to play it by ear, but they were stuck there until Tuesday. They ordered pizza and chicken wings for dinner and settled in for the night.

They quietly and carefully discussed the surgery with which they were going forward.

Andrea said, "Ya know, if there were only the conjoined twins, we wouldn't have a dilemma on our hands. We could just live out the pregnancy as long as they were able to survive. That's just not the case. Everything we're being told is when, not if, the twins die, then Thomas will shortly follow. How can it be right to just sit by and let that happen? I don't even want to think about these kinds of things."

Sean also realized the deadly situation they were in. The babies were even rarer than anyone realized. They couldn't separate shared vessels, because theirs was not a standard shared placenta. What happened went against everything the experts knew. All statistics showed that in order to have Twin-Twin Transfusion Syndrome, the babies *must* share one placenta. Well, that simply wasn't the case. They actually had two placentas that were fused together. It was as rare as could be. Then, in addition to that, they ended up sharing vessels back and forth through the two fused placentas. Even the thought of them ending up with Twin-Twin Transfusion Syndrome was impossible!

It was a heavy, heavy burden to carry. When they first found out their babies were in trouble, they prayed to God for peace. They felt confident in their decision to move forward, because they believed that if God intended for them to go a different direction with a different plan, then He would have given them the gift of turmoil, not His calming peace. That is not to say that God intended for their babies to die. God doesn't cause death or suffering, but He does sift through the dirt in life and still allows some of it through. Sin is what caused death and suffering, and people will be facing the disastrous consequences of that sin until the day we die or the day of God's return. People are not being punished for their own sins just because God allows bad things to happen to them. If a person waits out the storms in life God will show them

expect a miracle   *51*

His plan even when it doesn't make sense at the time. They can't see the pot of gold from where they stand amidst the stormy waters; sometimes they can't even find the rainbow on the horizon, but it is always there if they trust God with all their heart, mind, and strength.

Despite their inability to comprehend fully how their situation could possibly be for the *greater good*, Sean and Andrea moved forward with the knowledge that God can turn all things for the good of those who trust in Him. And they believed God would definitely use those circumstances for Thomas's benefit.

On Monday, they slept in until nine fifteen and figured they should at least get up while breakfast was still being served. After the buffet, they went back to their room, kept the shades pulled, and slept until noon. Sean went swimming again while Andrea soaked her feet before getting a repeat lunch of cold sandwiches at the hotel lobby. They also bought a disposable camera to record these events, since neither of them had thought ahead to bring their own and Andrea was an avid picture taker. Andrea picked up a postcard with a picture of the Golden Gate Bridge on it and mailed it off to the people at work.

Early in the afternoon, Sean wanted to get outside, so they walked around the hotel grounds and down the waterline. Back in the room, Andrea needed to call the nurse back to verify an appointment for Tuesday. They found out they had a fetal echo scheduled for one o'clock the next afternoon. Andrea started to get nervous and uptight again about the fact that they didn't know what to expect after that night. The last couple of days had at least been predictable, although boring. The unknown was frightening to both of them. For dinner they ordered in more delivery. This time it was a hamburger for Sean, spaghetti and salad for Andrea, and drinks for them both.

## PSALM 57:1 NIV

Have mercy on me, O God, have mercy on me, for in you
my soul takes refuge. I will take refuge in the shadow
of your wings until the disaster has passed.

Tuesday was their big day. They knew everything would be changing from that day on. They ate their last buffet breakfast and pulled out the business card the nice cab driver had given them on Saturday. She was more than happy to come and pick them up and give them a ride back to the hospital. They found their way up to the fourth floor to have the echo done of the babies' hearts. Sean decided to call his parents while they waited and asked Andrea where his dad's cell phone was. She reached into her bag and it wasn't there. A panicked feeling came over them both. They searched in desperation with no luck.

Sean asked, "When was the last time you saw it?"

"I know I had it as we got into the cab," she said as she shook her head.

Sean pulled out his work cell phone and the card of the cab driver. Luckily, she did find the phone, and Sean went downstairs to meet her at the front doors. He kept wondering what the chances were that they would actually have the phone number of the cabby who gave them a ride. Pretty odd, he thought. Andrea felt stressed out by the phone fiasco because she was so used to having it all together. She was embarrassed and felt bad for causing the unneeded stress.

They were told from the beginning of the echo it would probably take about three hours! Andrea asked why, and they answered because of the three hearts there were to examine. She didn't understand what the reasoning would be to study the twins hearts so thoroughly when the decision had already been made to have the surgery that would ultimately end their

expect a miracle   53

lives. She felt so heartless for saying that, but the fact was that they would only be tortured further by more detailed information about the twins. It was hard for Andrea to lie on her back for that extended period of time as well. She subconsciously didn't want to be studied for research purposes out of someone's curiosity.

After the man had done a detailed examination of Thomas's heart, he went to discuss it with the head of the department before continuing. His boss came into the room and looked for a few minutes at the twins' hearts himself. It didn't take very long for him to determine that, with a shared outer wall, the hearts wouldn't have the ability to function outside of the womb. He told Sean that they wouldn't put them through the entire echo of the twins.

They were sent upstairs for a meeting with Dr. Lee, one of the fetal surgery team members. He wanted to sit them down to discuss the procedure and appease any concerns they might have about what was going to happen. Both Sean and Andrea had a pretty general idea of what was planned. He shocked them by sharing that the surgeries they were performing were so new that, had their pregnancy happened even three to five years earlier, there probably wouldn't have been anything they could do to help. Andrea's life would be in great danger, as well as the babies.' The doctor explained the risks of having the surgery. There were the obvious risks to Andrea of any surgery, which were anesthesia complications, including possibly death. The major risk to Thomas was a stroke. At the time they cut the blood supply to the twins, there could possibly be a sudden blood pressure change to Thomas, causing him to suffer from a stroke. This could cause death, mental retardation, cerebral palsy, as well as many other possibilities. During the surgery, there would be a person in place who would be constantly monitoring his blood pressure and heart rate. It took time to get the surgery scheduled because of the magnitude of personnel involved in those types of procedures where there were two patients involved, not just one. They were sent to the nurses' station, where they were led to their room just down the hall. It was room 1518, and they were on the schedule for surgery at eight o'clock AM.

The nurse prepared all of the admitting paperwork and took tons of pre-op blood and put in the IV line. Andrea had dinner provided by the hospital since she was officially a patient now. Sean went downstairs to the cafeteria to get some dinner and brought it back up to eat with her. As they were accustomed to, Andrea was feeling queasy and, before they could prepare, she threw up red Gatorade all over her bedding. The nurse was quick to remove her sheets and bring new ones. She also brought some sheets for Sean, who had a chair beside Andrea's bed that unfolded to make a bed.

There was a fetal heart monitor on Andrea's belly all night, which made it almost impossible to get any sleep. They were both nervous about the next day and hardly slept a wink. Andrea couldn't have any food or drink after midnight to prepare for the morning to come.

### PSALM 55:1–2; 4–5 NIV

Listen to my prayer, O God. Do not ignore my plea. Hear me and answer me. My thoughts trouble me and I am distraught … My heart is in anguish within me; the terrors of death assail me.

### DEUTERONOMY 33:12 (TLB)

He is beloved of God and lives in safety beside Him. God surrounds him with his loving care, and preserves him from every harm.

Wednesday, July 3, was a day Sean and Andrea would remember for the rest of their lives. That day brought sorrow for lost

expect a miracle   55

babies, hope for an unclear future for one baby, and an entire flurry of mixed emotions about their future as a family. They were awake at seven AM to prepare for the eight o'clock surgery. Andrea was taken on a bed downstairs to the pediatric unit. They were taken in a service elevator used for the purposes of transporting patients and equipment. As Sean followed, Andrea watched the tiles on the ceiling go by, which made her feel sick to her stomach, big surprise. When they were parked in a small curtained area just outside of the operating room, Andrea asked Sean to ask a nurse for a vomit bin just in case. She brought one of those pink kidney-bean-shaped bowls, called an emesis basin. The ceiling and walls of that room were decorated for children with pictures of animals and fun, brightly colored things to take your mind off of where you were.

The anesthesiologist came in to talk to them first. He asked the usual questions about her history with anesthesia and any known medication allergies. He hooked her up to the IV line but didn't start anything yet. After he left the room, Sean noticed Andrea was still holding the little pink bowl in her hand in a position that almost looked as though she were waiting for someone to do something with it.

He asked her very seriously, "When are they going to get your ice cream sundae?"

They were still laughing heartily when the anesthesiologist came back and told them it would be just a couple of minutes more. That made Andrea suddenly nervous, and she looked into Sean's eyes suddenly as tears began to run slowly down her cheeks. He looked away for a short moment and said, "Don't do that, you'll get me going too."

Andrea prayed an earnest and heartfelt plea for Thomas's life. She asked, "God, please take care of the twins during this surgery. I just ask that You take them to be with You in heaven

andrea merkord

until the three of them can be together again with perfect bodies."

She believed it wasn't appropriate to pray for specific outcomes, because it may not be God's plan. It was best to just pray for everything to turn out according to His will. She had always stuck with that, until that day.

She continued, "Please be in the operating room with us and take care of Thomas. Keep him well and healthy. I want You to hold him and protect him *in Your hand* during the entire surgery."

It was the first time she had made such a demand of God, without following her request with "Your will be done." She didn't remember Sean kissing her good-bye before he watched her being wheeled into the room down the hall where he wasn't allowed to follow. All he could do was go back to the maternity ward and wait for any news of the outcome.

Sean soon discovered Andrea's hospital bed was ten times more comfortable than the foldout chair he was sleeping on. As he passed the time, he was flipping through the channels and eating the breakfast he picked up in the cafeteria downstairs before returning to the room. Time passed very slowly as he continued to channel surf.

A few hours later, the nurse came into the room and said, "I have some bad news. You'll have to give up the bed. Andrea's coming back."

Sean was scared by the beginning of her statement and quickly breathed a sigh of relief when she finished. He quickly jumped off the bed, and it was taken downstairs to transfer Andrea to it for her ride back up to the fifteenth floor.

Andrea could hear Sean's voice before she opened her eyes. He was telling her that the surgery went well and something about the blood pressure to Thomas. He was also the first person she saw when she opened her eyes. She tried to swal-

expect a miracle  *57*

low and realized her throat felt like a chalkboard. She hadn't thought about having a breathing tube down her throat during the surgery. The nurse handed Sean a small Dixie cup full of little round ice cubes. Andrea sucked it down fast and immediately asked for some more. Sean was shown by the nurse where to get more ice and drinks for both of them. For the rest of the day, they had a nurse totally dedicated to Andrea's postsurgical care. With two straps around her belly, she was being monitored for contractions and Thomas's heart rate. With the babies only being seventeen weeks gestation, Thomas was so small and mobile that it was nearly impossible to keep him on the monitor for anything but a couple of minutes at a time. Andrea wasn't allowed to get up yet and couldn't delay the need to use the bedpan, not once, but twice before she could get up and walk. She was complaining to Sean how it was the first time she had ever used a bedpan and how embarrassing it was to have the nurse take it away. He told her that he had talked to the nurse before Andrea was returned to the room after surgery and they were debating about whether she needed a catheter or not. Andrea was horrified at the thought of anything like that, and she would have had a conniption fit if she had woken up with one! She was the most private person when it came to the intimate parts of her body, almost to the point of extremes. The first thing she noticed once she was fully awake from anesthesia was her underwear had been removed.

She looked at Sean and asked, "Why are my underwear gone?"

He laughed and showed her the small plastic baggy they had discreetly placed them in for her labeled BIOHAZARD. Sean thought it was so funny, he felt the need to take a picture of it for safekeeping.

Andrea was made fun of at work for being so paranoid about her butt. Her saying was always, "Butts are private!" Trisha thought it was great to walk by and hit her on the rear end with empty boxes and say, "I touched your private butt," or "I touched your butt with my box."

Trisha was a character to spend all day with and Andrea was missing her.

While Sean was having burgers and pizza from downstairs, Andrea was thrilled to have her first meal, even if it was in pure liquid form. After eating, or rather, drinking her tea, bouillon, and Jell-o, she was feeling sick to her stomach again. Andrea told the nurses she was on a prescription for nausea but had run out of it and had none to take. The nurse got the prescription from the doctor and gave her the choice of a pill, an injection through her IV, or a suppository.

*Hmm*, she thought, *tough choice*, "How 'bout through the IV."

The instant dose of it made her feel lightheaded and a little loopy. She took a short nap while Sean watched TV.

Throughout the night, the nurse was in at least every hour to monitor the baby, since he wouldn't stay in place. The machine printed out a continuous feed of paper so the doctors and nurses could come in and look back at the previous time period. At one point, since they couldn't get a long strip to watch on him, the nurse stayed at the bedside for fifteen minutes holding the monitor in place with her hand and keeping his heart rate on it so they could get some sleep and she could get other things done. She thought it was unrealistic for the doctors to expect a fetus that small to be able to be monitored continuously.

Independence Day came, literally, and Andrea was finally able to take a shower. She felt great and even did her hair and make-up. The nurse even commented after her hair was clean, "Wow, there's blonde hair under there after all."

Andrea had a maternity shirt perfect for that day with an

American flag waving across the front of it. Flag shirts of all sorts had become the fashion of the year after the Twin Tower attacks of September 11.

They were sent downstairs for an ultrasound to check how the surgery had gone. Watching the monitor was different now knowing the life of their two twin babies had been ended yesterday in an attempt to save the life of one. Was it a fair trade? Nothing in that entire circumstance was fair, to Sean and Andrea, to the twins, or to Thomas, who could suffer irreversible damage because of what they'd done. What would it be like to live knowing that two died to save one, and you are that one? Would Thomas spend a lifetime trying to live up to the expectation created with the need to prove he was worth the sacrifice?

After returning to the room upstairs, they met with Dr. Weiss to discuss the findings of the ultrasound. She was a short young woman with wavy, dark hair. She repeated the information Sean already had heard. Thomas's blood pressure was stable during the entire procedure. That morning's ultrasound showed the blood flow had stopped going through the cord, but there was still blood "moving" in the body of the twins. Not to be mistaken by blood *flow*, this was blood that was shifting with the movement of Andrea's body. The doctor told them that they really wanted to give it another day and check it again in the morning with another ultrasound. They had the option to go home if they really wanted to, which, of course, they did. They had already spent too much time away from home as far as they were both concerned.

Sean asked the doctor, "What would happen if there was blood still flowing?"

"I don't know. I'm not sure we would go back in to do anything about it anyway."

She left them alone to discuss between themselves. They

60  andrea merkord

both wanted to go home so badly, when she returned, she wasn't surprised at all by their decision to leave that day. She did request they return to the hospital later that month to have a fetal MRI done on Thomas's brain. It could show whether there had been any damage done during the procedure. Andrea took the appointment card from her with no intention of coming back. San Francisco would not hold happy memories for her and having an MRI wouldn't change anything for Thomas's future, so there was no point in having one.

The daunting task of finding a flight on short notice on the first Fourth of July following the 9/11 terrorist attack was left to Sean. There had been a shooting that morning at the L.A. airport, which made getting on-line flights impossible. Sean called his parents to check for some and call back. After just a short wait, they returned the call with no luck. They were desperate to go home, and their nurse, Chris, helped Sean make some calls to the airlines. Sean and his mom were trying airlines directly and both came up with ridiculously high prices. After Sean chased his tail for a while trying everything he could think of, Chris got on the phone herself with Alaska Airlines and got them a cheap quote, which Sean booked.

Andrea was thrilled when they returned to the room with a flight plan. She called her mom, who was spending the holiday by the pool at home, and asked her to pick them up in Portland that evening. Chris stressed to them it was important they get wheelchair escorts for Andrea at both airports. She wasn't allowed to do large amounts of walking and was supposed to take the next week off of work to rest and recover. She was also to make an appointment for the following week for a follow-up ultrasound. They were discharged and waited downstairs at the front doors for a cab.

It was cold and windy outside, and Andrea began to shiver. There were two sets of automatic doors going into the hospital,

expect a miracle   61

and she decided to stand in between them to protect herself from the wind. Sean had on shorts and was waiting outside with their bags. It seemed to take a long time for their cab to arrive, so Sean called them again. He was told it should be about five more minutes. After what felt like fifty minutes, they were on their way. The driver was a tall, middle-aged black man, who was very talkative and friendly. Almost excessively so. He asked them what they were doing in San Francisco, and they gave him a brief synopsis of their last week's experiences.

He could hardly believe it was true and kept asking, "You started out with three babies? Were you on fertility drugs?"

"Nope. Everybody we talk to asks us that."

At the airport, they checked in their bags, and there was a wheelchair escort for them there. It was a long walk down to their gate, and the girl who was pushing Andrea chattered the entire way about terrorist attacks on airports. They were happy when they finally reached their gate, and they told her thank you and good-bye. The flight was pretty empty, and they were both tired. It was the first flight Andrea had ever fallen asleep on, but she awoke when they were getting ready to land.

Coming off of the plane in Portland, there was also a young girl there ready with a wheelchair for Andrea. She wasn't quite as talkative as the previous escort, but it was wearing on them anyway, because it had been a long day and the flight was late. They hadn't taken off on time because there was a man who had checked baggage onto the plane but had never boarded. They had to remove his bags from the baggage hold because of the risks of bombs being planted.

They were taken all the way downstairs to the baggage claim and went back upstairs to meet their ride. Andrea had gotten confused, and they realized they were actually supposed to be downstairs to be picked up, so they went back down again. Amber, who lived in a suburb of Portland, had come to pick them up. She drove them the first hour South on I-5 and they stopped in Wilsonville to meet Mary, who had been joined by April, who was dressed neatly in a darling striped maternity shirt that really showed her round belly.

Before getting back on the road, they decided to stop and get some snacks. They all had a taste for something different. Being directly off the freeway, there were plenty of fast food joints from which to choose. They headed toward Burger King and Taco Bell, then someone mentioned Wendy's, so they headed that direction. While heading toward Wendy's, Andrea saw a Dairy Queen sign and that was it. Ice cream sounded good to everyone.

Sean and Andrea intended on going home that night, and just crashing once they got there, but by the time they reached Steve and Mary's, they knew neither of them had the energy to keep their eyes open for the two-hour drive in the dark. After taking some pictures of the two pregnant sisters, who were much closer in size than they should have been, April went home. Mary asked if they were going to stay and made up the day bed for them in the small spare bedroom next to hers. She had given them the option to sleep out in the big bed in the outside room. That was the room Andrea had during high school. It was separate from the house and connected to a very large garage. The room measured twenty-four feet by twenty-four feet. Since the girls had all moved out, it had become Steve's playroom. He had a TV and computer and all of his Ham radio equipment, which had become his latest hobby. They decided not to sleep out there because it smelled so badly of smoke, so they slept in the smaller bed in the house.

Steve and Mary had to work on Friday and were both gone when Sean and Andrea awoke in the morning. Roger and Bobbie's fifth wheel was there, so before leaving, Sean and Andrea went out there to visit her grandparents. Grandpa had

expect a miracle   63

answered the door and invited them in. Bobbie wasn't there. She'd had to fly down to California, where her daughter was going through a lawsuit against some doctors who had failed to diagnose her skin cancer. It was great to visit with Grandpa, and he was emotional just imagining what they must be going through. After a short visit and some cold drinks, they hit the road.

On the way home, they stopped in a tiny town on Highway 22 called Gates. There was a Mexican restaurant they decided to try for lunch. It appeared they were the only customers and their server was about eleven years old. The food was okay, but nothing to write home about. As they were driving down the highway, an old Lionel Ritchie song came on the radio. It's so easy to tune out songs that are playing in the background of life. Music had always been such a big part of Andrea's own life and specific songs could always help her *remember when* ... This was another such song. When she heard the words "Thinkin' about you, baby, just ... blows my mind," parts of the song saying words like "Thank you for staying," Andrea began to cry, and Sean wasn't sure why. She was so relieved that Thomas was still with them on this ride back home. They had been so afraid they would come back from San Francisco without him.

### ROMANS 8:18 NIV
I consider that our present sufferings are not worth comparing with the glory that will be revealed in us.

It felt great to get home after being gone so much longer than they had planned. Hanna was at the door to greet them and to tell on Trisha for what she did to their home while they were away. She and Elizabeth knew their lives had been turned upside down and they both, along with Leah, spent the previous Saturday morning cleaning their entire house from top

andrea merkord

to bottom. There was a drawing and a note from Leah, and Andrea nearly cried. The couple couldn't believe what great friends they had, who would go out of their way on their weekend off of work to clean their home. Of course, it was a chance to get together and go shopping afterward!

Sean and Andrea spent all of Friday afternoon sleeping. Over the weekend, they unpacked their bags and completely vegged out, happy their ordeal was behind them. Maybe now they could just pretend that they were just like other couples and continue on with the pregnancy normally.

Andrea had the nerve to say to Sean in private conversation, "I believe people are tested throughout their lives with difficult circumstances, and I know we just were, but it was much easier than I would have expected it to be."

They both agreed that another couple, without faith to fall back on, would have had a much tougher time of it. God had answered their prayer for peace in their time of distress. That was the biggest gift they could have been given.

Looking back on the past two weeks and how much had transpired, Andrea realized she hadn't cried very often, which wasn't like her at all. She was the type of person who would cry at Kodak commercials. Maybe there is an internal defense mechanism that kicks in when people have no choice but to face the hand they've been dealt head on. That's just what Sean and Andrea had done. They were proud of the way they had handled it and were confident they had made all of the right decisions.

### 2 CORINTHIANS 13:6 NIV

And I trust that you will discover that we have not failed the test.

# PEACE FOR DESPAIR

**PSALM 34:18 NIV**
The Lord is close to the brokenhearted and
saves those who are crushed in spirit.

*A*fter breathing a huge sigh of relief, Sean and Andrea were ready to move on and rest their hopes on this one precious and amazing life remaining inside of her. The body of the twins would remain inside until delivery. The term the medical people used was "resorbed." The body would deteriorate and basically become partially absorbed by the time Thomas was delivered. Doctor's never mentioned giving the parents the chance to see them and say good-bye; there would be no point in that. They would be barely identifiable with the large amount of time passing between the date of their death and the date of the delivery.

Sean liked to think of the twins as Thomas's guardian angels. He would discover that he was oh so right. Nearly three years later, Andrea felt an overwhelming urge to name the twins and chose two of their other favorite choices, William and Andrew. She found an old baby name book by complete accident one day and looked up those two names. What she discovered blew her mind. Andrew meant "brave" and William meant "protector." Truly, God given names.

What an experience to share with people he would meet. How his life began with such a rare situation and almost no chance of a future. How many other people would have chosen to throw up their hands and end the pregnancy, deciding too soon there was no hope there? Although the ethical dilemma was one no person should ever face; does one watch all three die or attempt to give one a small chance?

Sean and Andrea felt, not comfortable, but satisfied with the decision they had made. It was a *life-saving* surgery. It wouldn't be until years later that they would have the opportunity to grieve the loss of the twins. Because they died at only seventeen weeks, there would be no death certificate issued by the state of Oregon. If they had been twenty weeks, it would have been different. Andrea wished there had been some public acknowledgement of their death, instead of just Sean and Andrea's private pain. That might have brought more closure at the time it was needed.

Andrea's biggest heartache laid in her wish that she had been given the chance to enjoy the thought of her children before discovering they were dying. If only they had been given an opportunity to treasure the idea of identical triplets and what life would have been like with them; to be happy about their pregnancy news and not mortified. She felt like the twins weren't done justice because they, in complete innocence, became the enemy of Thomas's chance at life.

Throughout their time in California, Sean had been fighting an ever worsening ear infection. It had become unbearable, and in the middle of the night on Friday, Sean drove himself to the emergency room. They administered heavy antibiotics and told him he let it go so long that he could have lost his hearing. Andrea received a phone call at two o'clock in the morning from a nurse in the ER. She needed to give Sean some pain medication, but he couldn't have it unless he had a ride home. Andrea crawled out of bed and drove her screaming body to the hospital around the corner and picked Sean up. The two of them were a sorry sight, completely exhausted, and in need of a great deal of rest.

expect a miracle   67

Trisha had left the mail that piled up for them while they were away, and Sean was concerned at the sight of an envelope labeled IRS. He slowly opened the letter and discovered that they owed good 'ol Uncle Sam another six hundred dollars on top of the six hundred they had already mailed out. Andrea had taken a deduction on their forms for which they didn't qualify. Oops! That was the last thing they needed at that time, but it wasn't the worst news that came that weekend. Tony and Carol had the unfortunate duty of telling Sean his twelve-year-old dog, Misty, had run away on the Fourth of July because of the fireworks and hadn't returned. They would never find out what happened to her, because she disappeared forever.

Going against medical advice, they both returned to work on Monday morning. Andrea already felt bad leaving unexpectedly for so long. John had new employees, and it left Trisha alone to answer all of the questions up in the office. Upon her return, Andrea was greeted with hugs from her friends, at least the few who knew the private details of her latest experiences. She told the manager, Steve, she couldn't do her normal duties and needed to take it easy as much as possible. He asked if she should even be there, and she said she wanted to help. The least she could do was data entry. All she would have to do was sit at a desk. For the most part, that's what she did. John received all of the lens shipments in Andrea's place. He didn't treat it as an inconvenience, even though, as the owner, he had bigger things to do.

On Tuesday, when Trisha went out to get the mail, she was excited to find the postcard Andrea had sent. There was the picture on the front of the Golden Gate Bridge. They could only laugh at Andrea getting there before the postcard did. That's mail in Central Oregon!

When Sean went back to work, everyone had lots of questions and were very concerned about them. He told them how

andrea merkord

the trip went and that everything should be fine now. His boss, Mary, from the Portland main office, was very glad for them that it was over.

That Friday, July 12, Andrea went to St. Charles Medical Center in town to have a follow-up ultrasound, by herself this time. Mimi saw her again, which was nice, and Andrea told her how things had gone. She still saw a tiny bit of blood moving in the body of the twins, but it was getting less. She did a few measurements of Thomas and took a good look around. She pointed out to Andrea an area of concern. There was a long stringy membrane floating in the fluid. She had noticed the dividing membrane between the two sacs was no longer intact. There was one big sac now, and Thomas was taking up as much room as he wanted. They had all been joking about how, with all of his fluid, Thomas had his own Olympic-sized swimming pool in there. After the fluid reduction, they joked he wasn't going to be happy about it being taken away.

Andrea thought, *Well, I guess he decided to take care of that problem himself.*

She called Sean when she got back to work and told him the latest findings.

"So what does that mean?" he asked.

"I have no idea. Dr. Davis wasn't sure what it meant, so if it's something to be concerned about, she'll call us later this afternoon at home."

Sean said, "Great."

She could almost feel him rolling his eyes as he said it.

Trisha was asking all about it, and Andrea had a seat in the cushy chairs at the front door to their office.

All Andrea could say was, "This could mean nothing. It could mean everything. I don't know." She just shook her head.

Dr. Davis never called back that evening, and they were

expect a miracle 69

left wondering all weekend again what they were going to do. They made the appropriate phone calls to family to give them the latest update.

The next week, Scott, from the Boise lab, was in the Bend lab to make some changes and see how things were going. Trisha and Andrea had come to really like Scott. He was a lot like John in his laid back nature and joking personality. It had become a custom whenever he was in town that Andrea and Trisha would take him out to eat somewhere. The last time he was there they had eaten at Shoji's. It was a fun oriental restaurant where they made your food on a flaming grill in front of your table, all the while making jokes and pretending to spill food on customers.

They decided to go see the new movie *Signs* with Mel Gibson. Andrea, Sean, and Trisha met up at the theater with Scott. Elizabeth went home to pick up Leah and they came also. Nobody expected the movie to be as scary as it was. Watching it in the theater probably assisted in the added drama though. Trisha spent the entire time with her feet up in her chair and her face in Leah's shoulder. Scott was sitting at the end of the row by Sean. There was a woman who sat in the one remaining seat next to him, and during scary or jumpy moments, she would jump and elbow Scott in the side, making him even more jittery. That movie touched an unexpected nerve in Andrea's heart. Who would have thought a sci-fi movie about aliens would have a deep underlying message?

Mel Gibson played a former minister who became angry at God for the accidental loss of his wife and felt that he had lost his faith. Through many of the events in the movie, he regained his faith and determined there are no accidents in life. Everything happens for a reason. Andrea walked away from the evening with a lot more than just a fun time with friends.

## JEREMIAH 29:11 NIV

For I know the plans I have for you," declares
the Lord, "plans to prosper you and not to harm
you, plans to give you hope and a future.

That week, Dr. Davis told them it would be best to go back up
to Portland and have the membrane looked at by the specialists. The couple felt horrible because they had to go back to
their bosses and tell them they needed to take Friday off to
head back up to Portland.

Sean had been trying to sell their Waverunner for the past
three months and received a call from a guy in Vancouver, just
over the bridge from Portland. Sean offered to bring it with
them to the appointment if he was serious about buying it.
The guy agreed and made arrangements to meet them there
on Friday. Sean thought it would be great timing to sell the
Waverunner with all of the new medical expenses they hadn't
anticipated. They really needed to sell it.

They rode back over to Albany to stay with Tony and
Carol again before the drive up to Portland Friday morning.
Sean asked Tony if he wanted to come along for the day, and
he was excited about joining them. Tony had never seen an
ultrasound before. Sean and Andrea, on the other hand, had
already seen more pictures of their unborn baby than most
parents see in a lifetime. Early Friday morning, they were on
the road again. They repeated the entire registration process
and sat in the waiting room of the diagnostic center for the
ultrasound. During the check-up, Thomas was rolling around
like a little party animal, and the lady actually had to stop trying to measure him and just wait a couple of minutes for him
to slow down. It made everyone laugh. The ultrasound proved
to confirm the situation with the divided membrane, but not
much more. Sean and Andrea could easily see the babies' parts

expect a miracle   71

and took for granted Tony could also. When the technician pointed out the profile and Tony asked her to be more specific, they realized that they had already become pretty good at seeing what she was measuring and checking out without any dialogue. It felt great.

The day would be another drawn-out set of visits with long waiting periods in between. After waiting a while upstairs in the waiting area of Dr. Di Federico's office, with a sense of déjà vu, she finally arrived. Tony waited outside while they went into the office to discuss the new information.

The doctor gave them both a hug and said, "Well, I was hoping I wouldn't see you guys again."

She went on to explain that the new condition added a large number of risks to the pregnancy. As if they hadn't already faced obscene difficulties. The blood in the twins was just about gone. The new risks were, now that the babies shared one big space, their cords could get entangled. In addition, the loose ends of the membrane could wrap itself around Thomas's cord, cutting off circulation. The baby was way too early to deliver at that gestational age, so there wasn't anything that could be done about it. They could only stand by and wait with baited breath.

The earliest time that delivery would be possible was at twenty-four or twenty-five weeks. That was a month away. It felt like an eternity to have to sit and wait while their baby could be inside dying. Dying inside Andrea's own body and there's nothing she could do about it. They still faced a fluid problem. It was still big and could cause premature labor. The doctor said they might need to do another amnio reduction as well, maybe more than one.

The course of action at that point was to go in for weekly check-ups and bi-weekly ultrasounds until twenty-four weeks' time.

From that point on, they would go in for weekly "non stress tests," or NST's, until the end of the pregnancy or until something turned for the worse. At these visits, Andrea would go to see Dr. Davis and be hooked up to a monitor that would record Thomas's heart rate for about forty minutes at a time. If something was going wrong, it would show in his heart rate, and they could deliver him early if necessary. Andrea wondered, *What happened the other* 10,040 *minutes of the week?*

With another heartbreaking situation to ponder, they returned to Albany for the rest of the weekend. Of course, the first course of action was to call a member of each part of the family and friends to resume the chain of never-ending phone calls that would continue to plague them for the long future to come. Sean couldn't believe something so simple could mean total disaster after what they'd already been through to save their baby.

Upon returning to Bend, the unknown future felt like a cloud hovering over their heads. Andrea returned the following week to see Dr. Davis, and she held her breath when the doctor put the handheld monitor on her belly to listen for the heartbeat. It was strong and steady, and she let out her breath with relief. Since the following week she would be having an ultrasound at the hospital, she made her next appointment to see Dr. Davis in two weeks.

In the meantime, Andrea was trying to enjoy her new found roundness. They were more than halfway through the pregnancy, and it should have been a time of excitement and joy. Instead, it was a time of fear and uneasiness unlike anything either of them had ever experienced. In her heart, Andrea quietly felt that things would end up okay in the long run. Ever since she prayed before the surgery and asked God to hold Thomas in His hands, she felt a calm, indescribable peace. She was not, however, a blind or naïve person. She knew it was

expect a miracle    73

God's choice to take him or leave him. Bad things happen to good people every day. It was that reality that kept the fear in her mind every minute of every long, excruciating day until the next ultrasound.

At work, friends and coworkers didn't know what to say. They knew each day was long and trying and mentally tearing them down. Family members continued to remain positive in their support, saying things were going to work out just fine. Andrea was talking on the phone to her mom one night, and she was walking around in what was supposed to become Thomas's bedroom. She looked at all of the bedding, the stroller and car seat, playpen, rocking chair, wash cloths, clothes, tiny socks, toys and rattles, story books, bibs, blankets, and even the diapers, wipes, and rash ointment, wondering if they were going to have to return it all to the stores. She complained that all she wanted to do was remove it all from the packaging and wash it and put it away. Mary told her she was being ridiculous to leave it all alone and told her to do what she wanted to do, open them all if she felt like it. Andrea didn't feel like she was being unrealistic to face the possibility that those items might never get used and felt like Mary was being a little naïve herself.

The next ultrasound finally came at twenty-two weeks. It was the beginning of August, and Andrea went to the appointment alone and was happy to find that Mimi was doing this check-up with her again. It was great to be with someone who didn't ask a million questions about fertility drugs and the like. Thomas looked great, and the membranes were still floating around in a world so far out of reach. They were relieved and could relax over the weekend a little bit easier than they had been.

Andrea was still taking the nausea medication and went to the grocery store to refill her prescription. As she was on her way, out, a lady asked her when she was due, and she told her December 9.

The lady gasped and stared at her with wide eyes, "You must have twins."

Andrea was caught off guard and didn't know what to say. Her mind swam for even one word or explanation to give, and when she came up with none after a long uncomfortable silence, she said, "Yeah, I do." She left quickly.

Pregnancy had been the total opposite of everything she had ever hoped for. It was supposed to be fun when people could finally tell you were pregnant and came up to ask you about it. Instead, all she wanted to do was run away from curious eyes. The last thing she wanted to do was discuss it with a stranger. Actually, the last thing she wanted to do was discuss it period.

At twenty-three weeks, they were finally getting used to the never-ending doctor visits. Many people in Dr. Davis's office knew who Andrea was when she got there. Her face was becoming a constant sight. The baby's heart rate sounded wonderful, and they were merely one week away from a more positive outcome. At least, the possibility of a better outcome if he needed to be delivered. Dr. Davis measured her belly, and she measured thirty centimeters instead of the normal twenty-three. They went out to the desk and had her nurse, Vicki, set up a series of weekly appointments beginning two weeks from that date. They started out with appointments through the entire month of September.

Every Friday, she could walk right in, tell Vicki she was there, and go to a quiet room that had a recliner in it. There she would sit attached to a monitor for about forty minutes and then she could leave. She had already planned to bring her headset and a book with her each time.

John continued to be patient and understanding with all

expect a miracle 75

of the appointments. Andrea tried to continue to be the speedy and productive person she had already proven herself to be. She felt guilty leaving all of the time, basically saying, "You have no choice about it, anyway." They were prepared for a long, drawn-out pregnancy of repetitive appointments.

### PSALM 31:24 NIV
Be strong and take heart, all you who hope in the Lord.

Twenty-four weeks came and changed their lives forever. From that day forward, Thomas would continue to be caught in a battle of life and death that would last well into the next year. The roller coaster ride that they thought had slowed down had reached the steepest hill of its journey and was just beginning its assent into the heights of uncertainty. The previous two difficult months they had just survived would prove to be a cakewalk in comparison to what they soon faced.

By herself, Andrea walked into St. Charles Medical Center for the fourth time on Friday, August 16. She was disappointed when a man came out to get her and found out that Mimi had gone on vacation. He got the rundown of her condition and got started with the check-up. He took a quick look at her chart, which laid out her complicated pregnancy, and read what he was supposed to be following up on. He did a quick check of the twins, probably out of curiosity to see for himself the rare phenomenon. At least, that's what Andrea thought in her mind. She almost felt a protective urge that she didn't quite understand. Even though they would never have seen life outside of the womb, she still didn't want her twin boys to be talked about or treated like freaks. They were babies, and more importantly, Thomas's identical brothers, whom he would never know.

Sean repeatedly told Andrea that he felt like the twins

were there for a reason. There was a purpose designed by God for things to turn out the way they had. Andrea felt like the situation probably came about on it's own through the strange events in nature, but God can make the best of anything this world presents as a problem.

Throughout the ultrasound, she watched as Thomas moved and wiggled around in the increasingly excess fluid, now sharing space with the twins and periodically coming into contact with them. It was hard to watch as his foot swung out and casually brushed them aside. When he was finished, the technician explained to her what he was seeing. He showed her the membrane where it attached to the side of the wall and followed it along into the sac where it had wrapped itself around a grossly swollen left leg. Thomas's left foot, which just happened to be right next to the other one on the screen, looked horrendous and swollen in comparison. She stared at the screen and shook her head in complete disgust. She could not believe this poor baby's luck and thought, *Here we go again.*

Going through a familiar routine, the head of the department was brought in to look at the findings and get some better pictures for the doctors to discuss later. They took measurements of blood flow going down to the foot, which looked surprisingly good considering the amount of constriction involved. As he walked her out of the radiology department, the man told her they had contacted Dr. Davis's office and she was on vacation, but another doctor from the office would be in contact with her soon. He put his hand on her shoulder and could only say he was sorry. She could see that he had no idea what to say.

He said, "I know you have already been through a lot. I'm sorry."

All she could get out was, "Not even once have we received good news," and bent her head down before turning to leave.

expect a miracle    77

On her way down the hall, it was nearly impossible to maintain her self control, which was very important to her. No matter how fast she walked, the hall felt like it was getting narrower and longer, like a scene in a horror movie. People passing by were a blur, and all she could think about was getting out. She was sick and tired of bad news. Her heart was in her throat, and she felt a scream welling up inside of her. All of the feelings she had held in through the entire ordeal were coming to a head. Before she reached the automatic doors and out of sight of passersby, the flood of tears came. She was practically at a jog when she reached the car, and very quickly, with shaking hands, opened the door and melted into her seat, dropping her head into her hands and letting it all come out.

It was a good thing that they lived two blocks away from the hospital, because she really couldn't see the road with the flood of tears that wouldn't stop coming. She immediately called Sean at work and through her shaky voice told him the latest heartbreaking news.

He wasn't sure what to think and asked, "Do you want me to come home?"

She said, "Yeah, can you leave?"

"I'll try."

When he got home a little while later, which felt like forever to Andrea, he gave her a big hug. They decided to go to his parents' house for the weekend again. Maybe he felt like he could escape it if they weren't home.

On the drive there, a man named Dr. Clark called, and the phone kept cutting out because they were past the mountains. Finally, Sean pulled off at a spot where the phone sounded clear.

Dr. Clark explained the risk of the new condition would be the foot could self-amputate, or basically cut itself off as Thomas continued to grow. They briefly discussed the risks of delivering him right away, which was the bare minimum gestational age they had been waiting for, hoping nothing would happen prior to that time. If delivered at twenty-four weeks, four months early, he would face an uphill battle that would most certainly lead to a disaster of some sort. Beside the fifty percent chance of death, he would deal with lung immaturity and brain bleeds, which could cause mental retardation, or commonly, the crippling disease cerebral palsy. The doctor told them that he would contact the Portland office again to schedule an ultrasound with the specialists.

The string of family and friend phone calls continued as they informed each of them of the latest development. Everyone had been holding their breath for the last four weeks, hoping not to hear any bad news. No one could believe it was happening.

"What are the chances?" The same question kept being repeated. "What are the chances?"

When Andrea was talking to Amber, she talked about the risks of having Thomas that early, and Amber said, "Then don't deliver him yet. Just let him grow and take the risk of whatever happens to his foot. Lots of people live without limbs just fine."

Without thinking about who she was talking to, Andrea blurted out, "I don't want a crippled child!"

Amber had a son with spina bifida. After hanging up, she felt absolutely rotten for what she had said and how she had said it. She never knew if it affected Amber or if she never thought anything of it. Nobody desires to have a disabled child, but life will deal the cards, and people have to do the best with what their given. Andrea was forced to begin thinking that maybe a child without a foot was better than no child at all. She realized how selfish she was being.

Sean spent the day on Saturday with his parents, and

expect a miracle   79

Andrea drove up to Salem to spend the day with Mary and April. They decided to go to Portland and do some baby shopping at Babies 'R' Us. Andrea didn't want to bring everyone down by dwelling on the stresses of her new situation, but the truth was, Mary and April were happy to be there for her at that time and hoped to lighten her load, if only for a little while. Andrea glanced at the preemie clothes, which she had never done before. She and April bought nearly matching winter outfits for their babies, both due that fall and winter. It was nice to buy something spontaneously in hopes for a future that was so uncertain.

They all went to the Clackamas Town Center and came across a store that sold music boxes. Everywhere they turned there were boxes of every size, shape, and color. April was doing her baby room in Noah's Ark décor, so she wanted to find a special box for her room. While Mary and April tried to narrow down which box April liked best, Andrea spotted a shelf across the room and went straight to a music box on a glass shelf exactly at her eye level. The box had a beautiful ballerina on it, which suited her, because Andrea had enjoyed dancing when she was in school. A profound and inspiring moment happened right then; when Andrea read the inscription on the box, she could hardly believe her eyes. Her eyes welled up with tears and she turned to where the other two girls were still inspecting Noah's Ark boxes. They were oblivious. Andrea knew that God had spoken to her that day through the message on the box in a personal and private moment. She kept it to herself, not telling anyone what had happened. At least, not yet.

### REVELATION 21:4 NIV

He will wipe every tear from their eyes. There will
be no more death or mourning or crying or pain,
for the old order of things has passed away.

Sean and Andrea returned to work on Monday only to tell their bosses and coworkers that they had to leave for an ultrasound on Tuesday in Portland. On Monday night, they drove back to Albany and up to Portland bright and early Tuesday morning. During the ultrasound, they could see how bad the foot looked. It was Sean's first look at it, and it was hard to absorb. The sight of it brought the harsh reality of the severity and precariousness of the new situation. Following the routine that had become the norm for them, they went upstairs to talk to Dr. Di Federico about the results of the ultrasound. As was also the custom, they were told to go and get something to eat and return in a little while. Instead of going to the cafeteria this time, they went directly downstairs from the office to a deli in the large, open atrium. They ordered sandwiches to share, and Andrea got herself a cinnamon roll, just because it looked good, and saved it for later.

Dr. Di Federico was sorry to see them back at her office. She thought they were such a nice couple and didn't deserve the continued drama that kept getting worse. There were only a couple of options.

1. Deliver him. Knowing the great risk of a baby his size, that was not a recommended course of action.
2. Call San Francisco. She could contact them and see if there was anything they could do to help Thomas out of his dire circumstances.

The last place they wanted to go was back to San Francisco. Not because of the hospital, but because their last experience there was not a good one. It was excruciatingly stressful and full of confusion, which is to be expected considering the reason they went. They told the doctor that they didn't want to

expect a miracle  *81*

go. They also knew that they had to give Thomas every option available to him, so they told her to make the call.

In preparation for a possible early delivery, the doctor arranged for Andrea to receive the first of a series of steroid shots to help Thomas's lungs develop. It was given to her by a nurse in the fattest part of Andrea's right hip. She grabbed a chunk of flesh and jammed the needle in so hard that Andrea flinched and held her breath until it was over. Another shot would need to be given twenty-four hours later. The best results of the steroids for Thomas wouldn't be until two weeks after receiving the injections. A person could be given up to three rounds of steroid shots, each two weeks apart if necessary or, more importantly, if time allowed.

It had been another long day at the doctor, and they were wiped out emotionally and physically. They prepared themselves for the three-hour drive back to Bend. On the way, all they could think about was how badly they did *not* want to go back to San Francisco. They secretly hoped it wasn't an operable condition. Immediately feeling guilty over putting their own desires before Thomas's well being, they could only wait and see what doctors in San Francisco said.

Back at work on Wednesday, Andrea could hardly concentrate. John held an office meeting to discuss the plans for organization of duties.

Andrea could only say, "Well, I may be leaving again any day."

She talked alone with Trisha for a few minutes about their options. Andrea told her it was a real possibility that Thomas could be delivered in a matter of days if his leg was in trouble and they couldn't operate on it. Andrea began to cry on Trisha's shoulder.

"Trisha, what if he dies?"

All Trisha could do was let her cry. Tears were falling

82   andrea merkord

on both girls' shoulders as Trisha attempted to take some of Andrea's pain away.

Trisha looked Andrea straight in the face and told her, "He's not going to die. He'll be fine."

They wiped away their tears and tried to concentrate on their work, as hard as it was.

Andrea decided to get out of the office for a few minutes and go to her favorite place for lunch, Subway. She always got the Subway Melt made the same way every time. It fit well into her regulated life. On her way back from lunch, with her sandwich in hand, she was mauled by Elizabeth, who said, "There's a Dr. Sandberg on the phone for you!"

Andrea ran into the office and sat down at her desk to get the phone. Taking a deep breath, she picked up the line. This time it wasn't as scary because she wasn't talking to a stranger. He sounded almost unnaturally excited and said they hadn't operated on an amniotic band in utero before and had been wanting to try it in San Francisco. They needed to get back down there as soon as possible. So that night they packed and drove back to Albany. This time they packed some warmer clothes and were prepared for about five to seven days.

### JOHN 14:1 NIV

Do not let your hearts be troubled. Trust in God; trust also in me.

Sean booked another on-line flight for a cheap price; unfortunately, the return flight was on Saturday. He booked it that way because number one, it was cheaper than booking two one-way tickets to San Francisco. Second, it was the soonest flight he could find. They learned from their last trip never to assume how things would go and knew they had no way to figure out which day they would need to get a flight home. All they could

expect a miracle 83

do was play it by ear. As hard as that was to do, they were fast becoming accustomed to it.

Tony drove them to the airport again on Thursday at about eleven AM. Their flight was scheduled to leave at twelve thirty. This time, when they arrived in San Francisco, they knew where they were going and were able to tell the taxi driver exactly. It was scary to be back because they were having more problems, but it was totally different, because they felt comfortable with the atmosphere and the hospital. They were even getting used to the fact that their lives were being played one moment at a time. There was no future to think about, because the future could change any moment. There was no "plan."

Whenever family and friends would ask them, "So, what's the plan now?" they couldn't answer. The correct answer to that question was, "There is no *plan*."

They checked in upstairs on the fifteenth floor maternity ward and were sent down to the third floor for an ultrasound at three fifteen. They were able to get a good look at the band around Thomas's leg. He still had good blood flow to the left foot, although it was quite swollen, but they were going to run out of time. At each ultrasound, they were reminded by the image of the twins bearing silent witness to the horrible tragedy of their rough beginning. There was always the sight of two little baby boys who would never know life on this earth with their brother. They could never forget it, nor should they.

Upon their arrival back at the top floor, they were put in an empty delivery room to wait for Dr. Sandberg to come see them. There was an immediate sense of déjà vu when they realized it was the exact same room they waited in the first time they were there; just a new situation. Sean lounged on the small couch again. Andrea paced about the large room. They had their luggage with them because they had no hotel reservations. The *plan* was to be admitted that evening for surgery the next day. After a couple of hours in the room, Sean was starving and told the nurse at the desk that they were going to the cafeteria for some food and would be right back up. They sat down to eat at a tiny card table in the room and the food hit the spot.

Five grueling hours later, at nearly nine PM, Dr. Sandberg finally came to see them. He had seen the ultrasound pictures and told them that the staff physicians thought it was worth trying. There would only be tiny incisions on Andrea's uterus. He warned them of the great risks of fetal surgery, which, they were well aware, included premature labor and fetal death. He had Andrea admitted to a small room around the corner, just one or two rooms away from the one she was in the last time. The nurse helped get all of the paperwork filled out. Andrea had planned for that part. She knew she would have to list personal belongings, such as jewelry, so she purposely left her wedding rings and necklace at Tony and Carol's house to be picked up on the way back home. Those were the three items she never removed, and she felt naked without them.

Inevitably, a short time later, the nurse returned to hook up the IV and take some blood. Andrea's fear of needles hadn't gotten better throughout the experience, and she could only hold out her arm and hold her breath. They always started by tying a loose piece of rubber around the arm to help pump up the veins better. Andrea had always been told she had great veins. The nurse was able to get a good one and, while Andrea looked the other direction and winced, she pierced the skin and shoved the needle in. She was applying pressure on the vein the needle was in and had a concerned look on her face.

She said, "I'm really sorry. It's in a valve. We'll have to do it again." With that, she removed the first IV.

Andrea couldn't believe she was going to have to feel that pain again. The nurse set herself up in another location and,

expect a miracle  *85*

with Andrea closing her eyes tightly, shoved in the next needle and hit her mark. She got it all taped in place and ready to be used for surgery the following day, which still hadn't been scheduled yet. The nurse pulled out another needle and a set of vials. She still had to take blood! Andrea could hardly believe her eyes and wondered to herself why she didn't take blood with the previous vein before hooking it up to the iv line. She was grinding her teeth together and holding her breath until it was over. She had always had a creepy feeling inside for a while after having needles poked in her, and she felt like she didn't want to move her aching arm. Dinner arrived, and Sean came back upstairs with his own dinner from the cafeteria, with which he was also already familiar. Andrea needed to enjoy her meal, because after midnight, she wasn't allowed any food or liquids. Sean's bed this time was different. The last time he had a cushioned chair that unfolded into a bed. This time he had a metal cot that he thought looked better for sleeping on than the chair did. He would find out he was mistaken. With his very large shoulders hanging off the sides of the narrow cot, he couldn't move without causing discomfort and could hardly sleep. Andrea had no complaints in her hospital bed, as was fair, considering she was the one going into surgery for the second time in two months.

Friday, August 23, nobody knew what time surgery would be. They were still trying to shuffle around schedules to accommodate this unexpected turn of events. All day Sean just hung out and wandered around the maternity ward. By the time lunch came around and they still didn't know what time she would go in, Andrea was finally allowed to eat something. A short time later, the couple was told they were scheduled for sometime after three o'clock. They both felt a little more nervous when they realized it wasn't much longer and they had to endure another frightening surgery with an uncertain outcome.

The anesthesiologist came to talk to them about having an epidural. Andrea wasn't sure she wanted one. She was afraid of the whole concept. Sean thought it was a good idea, but then again, he wasn't the one getting one. It would be given to her for pain management after the surgery and would make her much more comfortable, he assured her. She finally agreed to go ahead with it and he got himself set up. She turned sideways across the bed with her feet hanging over one side. The food table was pulled around in front of her and a pillow placed on top of it. The back of her gown was opened (leaving the top of her rear end exposed, which, of course, she couldn't get past in her mind), and he asked her to lean over the table arching her back like an angry cat for him.

He felt around between vertebras to find the right spot. He told her to be very still and hold on to the nurse's hands, but she held on to the end of the table instead while the nurse had her hands on Andrea's shoulders. Sean was curiously watching from the back, holding his breath in empathy with her. The first shot was for numbing and was very uncomfortable. Then he proceeded to place the epidural catheter, which would continually feed medication as she needed it after surgery. The line was taped all the way up her back and left easily accessible above her shoulder. She felt queasy and left her head lying down on the pillow for a couple of minutes.

While the man cleaned up, he got into a conversation with Sean about the fact that he was off to Hawaii the next day. That immediately helped the couple forget their current crisis for a split second. Sean told him they had gotten married in Hawaii on the island of Kauai, often called the Garden Isle. It was by far the most beautiful place either of them had ever been. They were married on a beach in Hanalei Bay. Andrea wore large-

expect a miracle    87

soled three-inch heels so she wouldn't sink into the sand, and Sean removed his shoes for the ceremony. Their little flower girl and ring bearer were also barefoot. It was a gorgeous day they would treasure forever. It was nice to think of such a happy time, even if it was only a momentary escape from reality.

Before she was to head to the O.R., the nurse helped Andrea put on what was basically a pair of white tights. They came all the way up to the top of her thighs. Apparently, she would need them later after surgery. She also told them that while Andrea was gone, they would be moving her to another room. Andrea was picked up by an orderly, who wheeled her on her bed downstairs to a different operating room area this time. They didn't go to the pediatric ward, but what she thought was the basement. Sean couldn't follow past a certain point and gave Andrea a big kiss with an overwhelming feeling that he had done this before. It wasn't an experience he had been hoping to repeat any time soon.

Once they were out of sight of Sean, Andrea felt the nervousness welling up inside of her. The last time, she didn't remember being wheeled into the O.R. This time she was wide awake. It felt like they were going down a maze of hallways and past a barrage of operating rooms. It was dizzying to watch the separate white ceiling tiles whizzing by over her head. The orderly slowed and then came to a stop. He was lost. After asking where O.R. four was, he switched directions and went straight there.

The surgeon welcomed her to the room at about three forty-five. As the anesthesiologist got her hooked up, he was quietly talking to her while the rest of the room was a blur of people. She felt him stick the little round monitors to her chest. He also put over her "tights" some plastic, cushioned straps that went from her calves all the way up her thighs. Once she returned to her room, they would be hooked up to a machine that would fill them with air, which would cause them to constrict and release, preventing blood clots from forming in her leg muscles while she wasn't able to move them herself. She was told that if blood clots were to form in the legs of immobile patients, they could travel to the heart and could even cause death. As if some magical wand pointed over her head, she was suddenly asleep.

Sean was excited when they moved their bags to a much larger room on the other side of the ward. It was obviously set up for two patients, and that meant Sean had a real bed for himself. No more cots for him. On this side of the building, from the large top floor windows, they would have a view of the bay and the Golden Gate Bridge. Off to the right, they could also get a glimpse of the Oakland Bridge. He was getting concerned when a few hours had passed and he had heard nothing of Andrea's progress. After being gone for three and a half hours, she finally returned to the room, much to the relief of her husband. She was still very heavily sedated and could barely hear Sean's voice telling her everything went great. All she heard was, "They gave Thomas shots ... They had to cut his leg ... " and she was out again.

They had a wonderful nurse named Winter that night, who took great care of them. When it was time for Andrea's suppository, she asked Andrea if she wanted to do it herself again, as she had before, but Andrea said, "I can't feel my body." Winter had to do it for her.

Andrea was absolutely mortified and said, "I'm so sorry."

Winter said, "Oh, stop it. This is part of what I do for a living."

When Andrea woke up on Saturday, she felt like a piece of all the many machines she was hooked up to. To her dismay, the incision on her belly was huge, not what she expected at all. It ran up and down through her belly button about four inches in length. She couldn't move her legs even if she concentrated with all of her energy, which made her feel creepy. Every few minutes she could feel the constricting around her legs by the mechanical air pump at the foot of her bed. To her horror, she realized she had a catheter in her bladder this time. Also, the epidural catheter continued to release pain medication. She had a blood pressure cuff around her arm that automatically took her pressure every fifteen minutes, and two different monitors strapped around her belly, one that measured contractions and the other to monitor Thomas's heart rate twenty-four hours a day. Through her IV line, she had standard fluids and magnesium, which was a tocolytic to keep her from contracting. Oh, and don't forget the suppositories every four hours!

The magnesium made her feel sick and queasy. It blurred her vision and made her feel extremely warm. She still wasn't allowed food but was finally able to chew on ice chips, yum! She never thought ice could taste so good. Getting out of bed was out of the question, so Sean had to keep filling her cup of ice chips for her. Luckily, the nurses reminded him of the code to get back into the room with the juices and things for patients to snack on. It hadn't changed since the last time they were there.

They had both been in contact with family and friends to tell them things went well. Andrea asked Sean to repeat the news from surgery since she didn't remember any of what he said to her the night before.

"You said they had to cut his leg?" she asked.

"Yeah. Your incision is big because they needed room to maneuver your uterus around. They had to give Thomas two shots to put him to sleep also. The band was so tightly wrapped around the leg that the doctor had to cut up and down across it to get to it. He said that when he did that, it literally snapped back in relief of the pressure."

Sean had been talking to his dad and asked if he wanted to come down and keep him company for a couple of days until they could get out of there. Around eleven thirty Saturday morning, he arrived at UCSF. Sean had met him downstairs and walked him up to the room. He walked in with his small, black rolling suitcase behind him and said, "Brushes for sale."

Andrea shook her head.

"Are you saying I need one?"

He came and gave her a hug. Since Sean had a bed of his own now, they used one of the unfolding chairs for Tony's sleeping pleasure.

The numbness in her legs was irritating, and Andrea asked the nurse if the epidural medication could be turned down. Later that afternoon, she had an ultrasound done, but this time they brought it to her. The man sat next to Andrea's hospital bed and did it there in her room. He was trying hard to be very careful of the large bloody wound running right down the middle of her abdomen, pretty much right in his way.

After the doctors had a chance to look at the ultrasound pictures, they came in to talk to them about it. Dr. Sandberg said the foot looked better, but it would be impossible to tell what the results would be until after he was delivered. There was another problem, however. It appeared there was another band that extended from the outside wall to Thomas's left arm. They would just have to keep an eye on it.

Sean just looked at Andrea and shook his head. "What did we do to deserve this? Is there ever going to be a day when we receive good news?"

They were both frustrated and disappointed that they

expect a miracle   *91*

couldn't catch a break. Andrea wondered if they shouldn't just deliver him and get the whole thing over with. Obviously, she wasn't doing a good job of carrying him. Maybe he would be better off outside. Tony got his first live glimpse of what they had been dealing with the whole time. It was highly volatile and unpredictable. No one really knew what it was like to be there. They could tell them over the phone, but to face it themselves is a different story.

Sean and Tony played a lot of card games and kept Andrea company with all of their joking around. It didn't take her long to figure out that Sean invited his dad down to entertain himself more than anything. She didn't mind though. Waiting around in a hospital wasn't exactly an exciting and uplifting experience.

Sunday, August 25, Sean and Tony ate at the cafeteria for breakfast. They were both impressed at what great food they actually had there. Andrea was just waiting for food of her own. She still wasn't allowed food but was finally allowed to have fluids. Her nurse that day wasn't by herself. She was training another lady who had been transferred from somewhere else. The trainee was a tall, young oriental lady who spoke with a strong accent. They stopped the magnesium and switched her to pills instead. She would take them every four hours. The epidural catheter was taken out, which Andrea was thrilled about. While the nurse was taking the Velcro straps off her legs, the trainee was trying to help and, without a word of warning, grabbed the urinary catheter and yanked it out. Andrea nearly swung her right leg out and kicked her in the face. Luckily, she was partly numb down there, but it was still an uncomfortable feeling. She probably wouldn't have been able to lift her leg that far anyway.

Sean and Tony ventured across the street of the hospital to a food court with a variety of options including, to their surprise, Krispy Kreme donuts. While they were away, Andrea was able to get out of bed and take a shower. The nurse helped her to stand on weak and wobbly legs. She felt like a newborn giraffe just learning to walk. They unstrapped her from the contraction and heart rate monitors and let her get her bearings. She first needed to use the toilet. Even the few steps to the bathroom door felt better each time. After shutting the door for privacy (remember, *butts are private)*, she bent her knees to sit down on the toilet. She immediately had to steady herself with the bar on the wall to her right when her legs nearly buckled beneath her. She almost fell straight to the ground. She giggled to herself, trying not to be heard by the nurses, who were changing her sheets for her, on the other side of the bathroom door.

As she got into the shower, she was more careful now that she realized the awkwardness of her weakened legs. She took the time to shave her hairy legs and wash and condition her hair. She didn't want to pack the salon-sized bottles she had at home, so she was using bottles from the hotel in Vegas they had stayed at the previous summer, the Luxor. They were drawn to its Egyptian design. It was the second time they had stayed there.

During her shower, Andrea remembered the first time they went to Las Vegas. They had gone with Sean's older brother, Craig, and his wife, Tandi. Their rooms were only a couple of doors away from each other. Sean was a late night person and Craig, the exact opposite. One morning, at about four o'clock, they passed each other in the hall, Sean just getting to bed and Craig just getting started. Andrea thought it was funny how each room had a phone mounted on the wall next to the toilet. She called Craig from that line, and when he picked up, she flushed the industrial sounding toilet and hung up the phone. She would give anything to be on vacation, anywhere but the

expect a miracle  *93*

hospital. This place had come to mean only bad memories for her. It wouldn't be something she treasured as an exciting time of her life, but the opposite—a place to remember the most horrible times of her life.

Sean and Tony returned with a box of Krispy Kremes and oversized smiles on their faces. While they ate their lunch of Subway sandwiches, which they also found across the street, Andrea was tortured. She was smelling the food of her favorite fast food restaurant. Tony also made the mistake of setting down his thirty two ounce Dr. Pepper a little too close to her. Sean saw the overwhelming temptation in her eyes and removed the obstacle before she could react. She was happy to find out that she was allowed to eat real food for lunch. This would become her favorite of the hospital meals. Sunday lunch was vegetable lasagna. It was absolutely delicious and hit the spot. She was feeling great, just a little sore at the incision site. It hurt when she laughed, which, was all the time with Sean around.

#### 1 PETER 5:7 NIV
Cast your anxiety on him because he cares for you.

With the beginning of the new week, the couple felt good about how things were going. Andrea was recovering well and could probably go home in a couple of days. She felt like a new person now that she wasn't connected to all of the equipment under the sun. It was down to the two standard monitors. The contraction monitor and the baby heart rate monitor both held onto her belly by the straps that wrapped around her waistline. She could only disconnect them long enough to go to the bathroom and plug herself right back in. Monday she was also taken off the suppositories, and she wanted to jump for joy.

Andrea needed another ultrasound and was taken downstairs back to the third floor. She was wheeled down on her bed and Sean and Tony followed. It was yet another dizzying trip watching the ceiling go by every step of the way. She felt really weird going down the hall in her bed, making all of the other people walking the halls move over for her. At least they usually took the service elevator for a more private, speedy trip back and forth.

The transport person parked her gurney next to the wall in the hall just outside one of the ultrasound rooms and took her chart into the staff. There were other people waiting out in the hall, and it seemed like the department might have been a little behind. While they were waiting, Sean overheard another couple talking about other fetal surgery patients. The woman was pregnant, and Sean heard them saying that there was this brave couple who had two surgeries and they first had conjoined twins complicated by Twin-Twin Transfusion Syndrome and had another surgery for the baby's leg. Sean knew it had to be them and walked over and asked about whom they were speaking.

They said, "Another couple that's here in the hospital."

Sean said, "That's us."

He introduced himself to them and they discussed their situation. They were also suffering from Twin-Twin Transfusion and had to choose between their twins to try to save one. The wife was crying and having a very tough time. It was difficult to see another couple suffer the same heartache they had so recently suffered themselves; but in a strange way, it was great to meet another couple who could relate to their own circumstances.

The ultrasound showed that the leg looked pretty good. The blood flow was an extreme improvement compared to before the surgery. It looked as though, for the time being, his leg and foot would survive. They looked around for the conspicuous

expect a miracle 95

band they had seen around Thomas's arm during the previous scan and said they didn't see it anymore. Sean would later tell Andrea that he still saw something there on the screen that looked like it was still connected to his arm.

There was also another concern they had. There appeared to be a very large blood clot in her uterus, and they didn't know whether it was hers or the baby's. It measured eleven centimeters! They would just have to watch it.

Since the IV had been in her arm for four days, it was policy to change it and replace it with a new one in another location. Andrea could only grin and bear it. The nurse got the needle in, and Andrea couldn't believe her ears when she said, "I'm sorry. I'll have to try again."

She couldn't believe it had to be done again, just as the first time the IV line was placed. Her luck kept getting better. Tuesday was a super day when they were told everything looked great and they were on track for being discharged on Wednesday. They spent the day playing cards and watching TV. Sean and Tony ate every meal at the cafeteria, or across the street at the food court, teasing Andrea with their great-smelling food. Sean would also look at Andrea's alternative menu every day and add choices on there for himself.

There was quite a bit to choose from on the alternative menu. It included plenty to drink, from colas to Gatorade. No Dr. Pepper though. There was soup, sandwiches, burgers, burritos, even ice cream bars. All she had to do was take her standard every day menu and write on any special item she wanted.

One problem they had was no airline tickets home. They had randomly chosen a flight just to get down there quickly, so they still would have to get another set of arrangements to return home. Before the surgery, they had been visited by the social worker named Stephanie. She was a very thin, middle-aged woman with dark hair and a wrinkled face. She came across as a hard, straight forward kind of person with what seemed like a New York way about her.

Stephanie had gone out of her way and contacted Alaska Airlines for them. She was trying to get the on-line tickets they had purchased to be exchangeable to another day of flight. She proceeded to tell the operator about Sean and Andrea's circumstances, and the lady on the phone started crying. She couldn't figure out a way to change the existing tickets. She offered instead to give them a pair of one-way tickets home that they could use any day with short notice in the next thirty days. She gave them authorization numbers to use when they needed to book the flight. Sean couldn't thank Stephanie enough for going beyond the call of duty.

They knew how fluid their situation was and wouldn't book the flight until they were 110% sure they were leaving San Francisco. They were finally learning to be prepared but to be flexible. There was no certainty in the near or distant future. Sean would wait until the last possible moment to book their flight home when needed, hopefully, the very next day. Fate would have other ideas though. The struggle that had brought them this far would turn to near disaster in a moment's notice. No one expected it to happen, and even the doctors didn't know what to think of it.

expect a miracle    97

# GLADNESS FOR MOURNING

**PROVERBS 3:5 NIV**

Trust in the Lord with all your heart and lean not on your own understanding;

Wednesday, August 28, would be yet another day to remember. Adding to a list of unforgettable moments in time, this day would soon be another mile marker down the road of Sean and Andrea's remarkable pregnancy and Thomas's unfathomable fight. They would be told by nurses Thursday that they just *knew* they were going to have to deliver Thomas that day, more than three months early.

They woke up with the *plan* of packing up and going home after a week in the hospital. It was about the amount of time they had anticipated, but they were more than ready to get back home. They had been told by doctors the day before that it would be necessary for Andrea to check into the hospital in Bend as soon as they got home. Dr. Sandberg guaranteed them that Andrea's water would break within the next two weeks. They needed to get straight home and play it safe.

As soon as he left the room, Andrea said, "Yeah, that ain't happenin,'" with a smirk on her face. "I have no intention of sitting in a hospital until December. We can't afford that anyway."

She figured she would do the same thing she did after the first surgery, which was to go back to work the next week. However, God would take care of those plans before she had a chance to destroy, through carelessness, all they had worked for. They had gotten that far by doing the right thing and they didn't seem to understand that Thomas wasn't out of the woods. Not by a long shot.

Andrea had gone to the bathroom early in the morning, as most pregnant women will do with a bladder the size of a pea. She was bothered by a tiny spot of blood on the toilet paper. She went over to Sean's bed quietly so as not to wake Tony and whispered, "There was blood, but I don't want to say anything because I want to go home."

Sean told her even though it was a tiny amount, which could be totally normal in another pregnancy, she probably should say something, but it was up to her. They didn't know it wouldn't make a difference either way. It would show itself later.

Andrea decided when the chief resident, Dr. Mannon, came in for her morning rounds, she would tell her about the blood. All Dr. Mannon said was, "I noticed you had a worried look on your face that I haven't seen before. It's probably nothing. I wouldn't worry about it."

That was that. Andrea was relieved. They were sent downstairs for a final ultrasound at ten o'clock. After that, Sean would book their flight home. There was a sense of excitement that this part of their journey was finally over. They would be given another chance to try to move on like normal. Or would they?

The orderly wheeled her down in a wheelchair this time, followed closely by Sean and Tony. An older man performed the scan, and he wasn't being careful at all. Andrea even gasped a couple of times when he scanned over her still fresh incision site without a thought for her comfort (or discomfort). She was getting very angry. He applied more pressure than she had

expect a miracle  *99*

felt during any previous ultrasound they had up to that point, which Sean figured was about sixteen different ultrasounds.

After sixteen ultrasounds, they didn't need explanations as to what they were looking at. It didn't matter, because it appeared to be the policy in San Francisco that the sonographer wasn't to discuss what they saw to the patient. It must be different everywhere. It would make sense, though, in a place where they deal with the highest risk patients, they don't want people speculating about what they see without the doctor's input. Everything looked great, and as soon as they got back upstairs, Sean was *planning* to call Alaska for their free tickets home.

They were placed out in the hall between some of the rooms to wait for their ride back upstairs. When Andrea lowered herself from the gurney down to the floor, they all noticed a big circle of blood on the sheet on which she had been lying. She went to use the bathroom, which was just a couple of doors down. The bathroom was located in a locker room area for the staff. There were lockers and curtains for privacy to the right and a handicap-sized bathroom stall to the left. She was still wearing a hospital gown and it also had blood on it. She couldn't sit down on the toilet without pouring out blood onto the floor. She tried to get herself cleaned up, but when she stood up again, the flood of blood came so fast that there was nothing she could do about it. She was totally oblivious to the possibility that it could be life or death in a matter of minutes. All she was thinking was that it was irritating that she couldn't clean it up fast enough.

A staff member came into the room and knocked on the stall. She asked, "Are you okay?"

Andrea said, "I don't know."

Sean was worried after seeing blood on the gurney and because she had been in the bathroom for so long. They were rushed back upstairs to the maternity ward, and her nurse was told what was going on. Andrea tried to use the bathroom in her room again and had to throw away the pair of underwear she was wearing because it was soaked. She was given a large feminine pad to wear, but it was overflowing in only twenty minutes time.

The staff got her hooked back up to the monitors that measured contractions and the baby's heart rate. The baby seemed to be doing fine for the moment, but Andrea was contracting quite a bit. She was placed back on the magnesium through her IV line in hopes of stopping labor from coming full force. The amount that she would be placed on regularly would be three grams per hour, but she was a started on a bolus of six grams in twenty minutes! She felt extremely hot and sweaty and totally out of sorts. Everything was blurry, and she was groggy. The day would forever be a total blur to her.

Because her condition had changed drastically that morning, she was back on bed rest with no food or drink. She would need to use a bedpan for the next two days and get help from the nurses to change the sanitary pads she needed. She was absolutely crushed that her situation had turned upside down again. They were so eager to be heading home, and now that would be impossible until the doctors could figure out what was a happening to her.

The large room she had been in was needed for other patients, and they were moved to one of the smaller, single patient rooms, since it appeared that she would be staying for a while longer. The doctors had discussed with them the possibilities of what might have been going on. The number one concern was placental abruption, which is when the placenta prematurely separates from the uterus. This can be deadly to the baby in a matter of minutes because it reduces or completely cuts off the baby's oxygen supply from the mother.

expect a miracle    *101*

Since Thomas's heart rate looked good and he didn't appear to be suffering, for the moment, any ill effects, they told them it could be a partial abruption. Part of the placenta could be pulling away. If that was the case, it could turn disastrous at any moment. Sean was completely worried and quietly pondering what that could mean for Thomas, and Andrea, for that matter. Andrea was barely conscious, in and out of sleep, and nearly unaware of their dire situation.

The room had a solemn and gloomy aura about it all day. Their nurse was wonderful and checked on them constantly throughout the day, making sure they were feeling okay with all that was going on. Without reassurance of even the doctors knowing what was happening, it was another ride into the terrifying unknown that they weren't prepared for. They just kept being taken by surprise time and again. They both wondered when it would all end. How could other pregnancies go off without a hitch, and yet they kept experiencing enough stress for a million pregnancies? Thomas was still fighting for his chance at life, and he wasn't about to be denied.

### ISAIAH 41:13 NIV
For I am the Lord your God, who takes hold of your right
hand and says to you, Do not fear; I will help you.

All day Thursday they hung out and waited. Waited for what? They didn't know. Andrea was still pouring out blood from who knew where. She was still on the magnesium. Luckily, it had been successful in stopping her contractions completely. The doctors had concerns that the blood might be Thomas's and scheduled another ultrasound downstairs. This time they measured blood vessels in the baby's head to check for anemia. Those tests came back okay.

After all other options were exhausted, the staff came to

the conclusion that it had to be Andrea's own blood. Although her blood counts continued to be at a normal level, there was talk of giving her a blood transfusion if it became necessary. When she called Trisha to give her the news that she wasn't coming home right away, the people at work could not believe Thomas's luck and wished them the best. After telling Trisha that they were talking about giving her a blood transfusion, she yelled over the phone, "Not in San Francisco!"

Andrea laughed and said, "I know! Oh my gosh, you read my mind. That's exactly the first thing I thought too. Aren't we horrible?"

They both laughed. It was amazing how just hearing Trisha's bubbly and girlish voice made Andrea's day one hundred percent better.

Sean got into teasing his dad about wearing the same shirt again and, after beginning to feel the pressure of the stay in the hospital, Tony took it personally and got crabby and uptight. Sean tried to explain that he was just joking.

"Dad, I'm wearing the same sweats as yesterday. I didn't pack enough clothes either. I was just teasing you."

Tony finished getting ready and quietly went downstairs to the lobby, where he usually found a newspaper to read for a while.

When they were alone, Andrea told Sean, "I don't need any more stress than we already have. He's supposed to be here to lighten our load, not add to it. Now you have to deal with his attitude on top of trying to keep me entertained and keep yourself from going into some stress attack. This is the last thing we need. If your dad can't handle it here, he needs to leave."

Sean left the room looking for his dad. When they met up, Tony apologized immediately. He admitted that the stresses were hard to handle, and he was getting claustrophobic in that tiny room they were in all day long.

expect a miracle  *103*

Sean said, "Dad, I'm not trying to be rude, but we don't need this right now. We have more on our shoulders than we can handle as it is. You've had just a glimpse of the ups and downs of our lives for the last two months. Welcome to my life. It sucks, but we have to be supportive and try to remain positive, as difficult as that may be."

After patching up a short-lived disagreement, they went upstairs and apologized to Andrea too.

Friday, since their situation hadn't worsened, she was taken off of the medication and allowed back out of bed. She was allowed to get up to take a shower and eat all of her meals. She was still bleeding huge amounts and had to let the nurse count the number of pads she was going through so they could monitor blood loss. It was disgusting and embarrassing.

When Dr. Sandberg came to check on them, not much had changed in her condition. He told them that it had been concluded that the blood was old blood from after the surgery. It was Andrea's own blood that had finally made its way down and out of her body. Since blood irritates the uterus, that is what most likely started the contractions she was having on Wednesday. At that point, it was reasonable to assume that, if the bleeding stopped, Andrea could be released to go home. She would have to be stable with no bleeding for at least a couple of days first.

Although things were stable, Andrea still needed to constantly have an IV in place. Since it had been four days again, it was time to change the location. No matter how many times she was stuck with needles, she never got used to it. It was a grinding chalkboard feeling every time that made her feel sick to her stomach. At least this nurse did a good job and got it over with quickly on the first try.

Sean talked to Andrea about the fact that he needed to be heading home and back to work. That weekend was the Labor

Day holiday, and he wanted to have an extra day to get settled back at home. She reluctantly agreed that he should leave on Sunday. He would be able to stay the night at his parents' house and head home on Monday. He would have Monday off of work and could get himself prepared for the return to work and life at home without her.

Her heart sank at the thought of him leaving her there by herself. What if she went into labor? He wouldn't be there for the birth of their son, who might have difficulties. What if something bad happened to Thomas and Sean never got to see him at all? She was also afraid of going through it by herself; aside from the fact that she would be all alone, in a different state, where they knew nobody, and Sean was too far away to visit regularly. She made him promise that no matter what happened, he would come back to visit in two weeks if she wasn't home in Oregon yet.

She said, "I don't care what you have to do or how tired you are. You book a ticket and get yourself down here to see me for the weekend."

She was hoping that time wouldn't come and she would be home by then. There were commercials on TV for their favorite reality show, *Survivor*. The new season started Thursday, September 19. She knew she would be home by then and they would resume their regular routines together. Every Thursday was *their* night. They would get in the truck and go through two drive thrus. Sean wanted Wendy's hamburgers and Andrea wanted Taco Bell. Then they would push the love seat together with the couch and prop themselves up with pillow and blankets to watch their shows together. They watched *Survivor* and then *C.S.I.* every week, set up with everything they needed for those two hours. Andrea fit perfectly on the love seat, and Sean got the couch. It was a special, fun time every week between the two of them; their "date night."

expect a miracle *105*

There was a library across and down the street from the hospital, so Sean and Tony went and used a computer to get on-line and purchase a plane ticket home for Tony. Sean got on a phone with Alaska Airlines and arranged to be seated next to him on the same flight. They were all set to head home on Sunday afternoon.

When they returned to the room, Sean was trying his best to mask his excitement. Andrea could see right through him though. She shook her head and said, "You could try to not be so excited to leave me here by myself."

With a sheepish grin he said, "What are you talking about?"

"I can see the happiness in your face. You couldn't hide it if you tried."

"I'm not happy to leave you here, but I am happy to be going home. I won't lie about that."

Andrea had a hard time on Saturday trying to forget the fact that Sean was leaving and just enjoy their last full day together. She tried to hide it, but her heart was already weeping inside in anticipation of saying good-bye. When the boys returned from the cafeteria after breakfast, they brought back gifts for Andrea. Sean gave her a beautiful vase of bright yellow flowers for her room, two magazines to read, and a book of word search puzzles, a journal and pen, and a mug and t-shirt that said UCSF on it. She thought, *Why would I want a t-shirt that says UCSF on it?*

He also brought something that she was surprised by. She was impressed at how thoughtful and sensitive he was to come up with such an idea. He picked out a beautiful card to leave on the board on the wall so that nurses and doctors who dealt with Thomas could write notes to him for when he arrived. The card read:

*106* andrea merkord

## BELIEVE

Faith can move mountains. Love unbreaks the shattered
glass; Believe with all your heart, my friend, and watch
the shadows pass. Everything will be alright.

Sean asked her if there was anything else she would like.

"The only thing I can think of is a certain book."

There was a series of Christian books she had been reading
and she hadn't purchased the latest one out, so they were on
the hunt. Their nurse for the day pointed them in the direction of the nearest bookstore. By the directions she was giving
them, it didn't sound very close for walking. It wasn't like they
had better things to do though. When they returned a while
later empty handed, Andrea was disappointed but grateful for
the effort.

That day was a special day. August 31 was Trisha's birthday. Andrea was thinking of her when a nurse rushed into the
room and stared at Andrea's monitor. She had been watching
Thomas's heart rate on the computer from the nurses' station
and it had dropped suddenly. The nurse was Chris, the same
one who had helped Sean find airfare home the first time they
were there in July.

She told Andrea to turn onto her left side, which apparently helps sometimes in those situations. There were several
tense moments as they watched the screen waiting for his
heart rate to climb back up to an acceptable rate. It appeared
to head in that direction, and Chris told her to stay on her left
side for a while and they would keep an eye on things from out
front. It put *another* damper on what they were trying to make
a good day. No one said much as they watched the monitor
with baited breath.

Suddenly, a small group of doctors and nurses ran into
the room and started messing with the equipment and straps

expect a miracle    *107*

on Andrea's belly. They were checking to make sure they were getting accurate readings. Thomas's heart rate had two more major dips and they told them what that meant. The resident explained to them that if it kept dropping down, they would have to perform an emergency C-section. They had all of the paperwork handy to have signed for an emergency procedure should it become necessary.

They had Andrea shift her position again. Hopefully, by changing positions, it could make things better. If Thomas was squishing his own umbilical cord, shifting his position could change things for the good. As the afternoon wore on, there were no more drops in his heart rate, and gradually they stopped holding their breath. On Sunday morning, they were told again by their nurse that they had thought for sure that Thomas was going to be delivered that day. He was having one close call after another.

Sunday was a hard day for Sean and Andrea. With the latest events being so fresh in his mind, Sean wondered if he would even get home before getting a call that Thomas had to be delivered. Andrea feared the same. She thought for sure that she would totally lose control when Sean had to go. When it came almost time to leave, Tony went downstairs early to give them time alone.

They kept looking at the clock, knowing that at one o'clock Sean had to go. Sean sat on her bed and they talked about how she would get along and that they would see each other soon. Sean left their video camera with her for that chance that she didn't make it home before Thomas arrived. Andrea hugged Sean with all of her might and didn't want to let go. He got up to walk away and she said, "No," and started to cry.

Sean sat back down by her and said, "You know I have to go," and gave her a strong hug. It was one of the most difficult things he ever had to do; walk out the door, leaving his preg-

*108* andrea merkord

nant wife in unstable condition in a hospital hundreds of miles from home. She watched him slowly close the door without turning around, which was probably best, and to her surprise, she didn't lose total control.

She sat there looking around the room, suddenly feeling very alone. She was sad to realize that there was nothing from home there with her. She didn't have any jewelry on, including her wedding rings. Not even a single picture of Sean. She had recently downsized her purse to an organizer that was much more compact and she hadn't put any pictures in it. Without much ado, she spent the rest of the day alone. Sean called during many stops along the way. He called from the San Francisco airport and the Portland airport. He also called from Albany at the Blockbuster Video they had stopped at and again late in the evening before bed. She really appreciated it.

There hadn't been very much bleeding through the night on Saturday or Sunday night, which was good. Sean called early Monday morning just to talk and again in the late morning before he packed up the car to head home to Bend. Amber called because she knew that Sean had left and that Andrea would be lonely.

It was a long, boring day between phone calls from family. In the early evening, she called Sean and they talked for a long time while he paid their bills. Even while they were dating, they had never spent much time on the phone together, partly because they never left each other's side for long enough to need a phone call. They had spent nearly every day together from the time they started dating. It was unusual for them to be apart.

#### HEBREWS 10:23 NIV

Let us hold unswervingly to the hope we profess,
for he who promised is faithful.

First thing Tuesday morning, Andrea was visited by Dr. Farmer, the surgeon who had performed the first surgery. She was accompanied by her residents doing rounds. Andrea wasn't currently her patient, but she stopped by for a quick visit. She asked how the bleeding was going, and Andrea told her that she was excited that morning because there had been practically no blood after the entire night. They talked briefly about how they would get her home if the bleeding did stop. A flight from San Francisco was only about an hour and a half to Portland, but then there's a three hour drive over the mountains to Bend. She could hop on a short flight to the Redmond airport, which would bring her twenty minutes from home, where Sean could pick her up. Just talking about going home had Andrea all worked up. It sounded like it was a real possibility in just a couple of days.

Andrea called Sean on his cell phone at work and told him what she and Dr. Farmer had discussed. Her phone call was cut short, though, by a nurse in to change her IV sight again. Yay! She also needed to give Andrea the second round of steroid shots. She got one that morning and would get another one twenty-four hours later. It didn't feel any better than the first time she got them. It really burned.

At eleven thirty, she was taken downstairs for an ultrasound. She was familiar with a lot of the people down there, but this lady was new to her. She was serious and didn't talk much at all. Andrea watched the screen as the lady tried to measure the areas of fluid around the baby. Since they always had a fluid problem, namely too much of it, Andrea was used to the whole process of measuring each quadrant for an average fluid amount in there. This time was different. Andrea could tell that on a couple of sides there wasn't even an amount to measure. When she finally found an area she could measure, the distance was so small that Andrea could tell something was wrong.

Back in her room, Dr. Sandberg and Dr. Mannon came in to talk to her. Dr. Sandberg sat down in the chair at the foot of her bed in the corner and Dr. Mannon stood nearby.

Dr. Sandberg said, "You have very low fluid now."

Andrea looked at them and said, "Yeah, I know."

He seemed very surprised or concerned about her knowing that information already and asked, "How do you know?"

"I was watching the screen, too, ya know."

He was rather curious that she had the ability to decipher what was on the screen. He told her that her water had broken. There was probably a leak that had been draining small amounts of fluid for a few days. It may have been disguised by all of the blood she was losing, and that's why she hadn't noticed a difference herself. Bottom line was that she wasn't going anywhere now.

She was immediately started on antibiotics through the dreaded iv line every six hours. Sean didn't have much of a reaction when she told him that evening. He remembered that Dr. Sandberg had guaranteed them it would happen sooner or later. He was, however, disappointed in getting more bad news. Now Andrea begged him to promise that he would visit in two weeks like they had discussed. He could only say, "We'll see."

Andrea began the domino line of phone calls with her mother. Mary said, "What?"

She had no idea that women could stay pregnant even after their water broke.

Andrea asked her, "Where have you been?"

She wished so badly that her mom would come down and spend some time with her, but Mary didn't feel comfortable taking time off work at her fairly new job.

Pondering yet another down spiral in their chain of events

**expect a miracle** *111*

was beginning to get a little too redundant. She could *almost* have a sense of humor about it. It was like a poorly written soap opera that was so ridiculous you would never believe it really happened to anyone.

When the head of the department, Dr. Laros, came to check on her, he plopped himself down in the chair and just shook his head like *what are we going to do with you?*

She asked him, "So, how long can a person go with their water broken?"

Dr. Laros said, "Now are we talking about a normal person, or are we talking about you?"

Andrea couldn't help but laugh. She had definitely been the exception to many rules. The mere unpredictability was what bothered her most.

"Most women, when their water breaks, will go into labor within twenty-four to forty-eight hours. You, however, could sit there forever. The longer you go without going into labor, the longer you can go after that."

He went on to tell her that what they would be watching most closely for with her was infection. With an open environment, there is a high risk of developing an infection that could hurt the baby. If that happened, Thomas would need to be delivered. She was given a chart to fill out every two hours. There was a thermometer by her bedside, and she was to chart her temperature throughout the day and night to watch for an increase that could indicate an infection. To make things worse, the thermometer was in Celsius.

On Wednesday, September 4, she was given the second steroid shot for Thomas's lung development. That was the second round of steroids she had been given, and Dr. Sandberg told her she wouldn't be given a third round. He really didn't see the need.

Andrea was still on the pills called Nifedepine that she was given every four hours to quiet any contractions that might come. On that day, her nurse had come in to give her the antibiotic that was on a six-hour schedule and gave her the Nifedepine too early. Andrea wasn't even paying attention until later when she realized what had happened. That threw her schedule off, which meant being woken up more times during the night to fix it, which, luckily the night nurse did.

Andrea was finally taken outside to a garden area in a wheelchair by an oriental lady who was part of the housekeeping staff. They sat out there quietly enjoying the fresh air and sunshine. It was a relief to get a change of scenery. She had been in that room for two weeks without a breath of fresh air. She was actually impressed that her nurse had realized that fact and made an effort to relieve Andrea's claustrophobia.

She had finally been given a piece of good news to share with Sean. Even though she had two surgeries, that didn't guarantee that a C-section would be required. She had the possibility, if everything went well, to have a normal delivery. That was wonderful news, because the last thing she wanted was another surgery.

Andrea tried to make sure she was writing in her journal at least every couple of days to keep everything straight. She had done a pretty good job up to that point. Since she had been there for two weeks, she went back in her journal to the day they had gotten there for the second surgery and labeled each day Day 1, Day 2, Day 3, and so on. This was day fourteen already. She also tried to use the video camera to update Sean on the latest, greatest excitement that he might be missing out on.

She set the camera up on her table and gave the audience the scan around the room. She narrated in detail each area of her tiny room with a good view outside and showed the monitor, which was still attached around her belly twenty-four

expect a miracle  *113*

hours a day to watch Thomas's heart rate. She could hear the pitter patter of it going all the time. It almost became comforting to her. Sometimes, when the night nurses would come in late to give her the medications, they would turn the volume down before leaving the room again. That really irritated Andrea, and she would reach over to turn it back up. She just thought, *Why would you do that? Don't you think if I wanted it turned down, I would do it myself?* They treated the equipment like some high tech system that was over anyone's head. There was an obvious volume button to use if you needed to. The frustrating part about it was that when she moved at all, sometimes the monitor lost Thomas's heart rate, and if it was off the screen long enough, the nurse would come back in and start messing with things.

It was difficult to have no privacy. Every time she got up to go to the bathroom, she would disconnect from the machine for a few minutes, which showed on the screen. She felt like a child at times. Sentenced to bed except for a brief time disconnected from the straps around her waist so she could take a shower.

Every day she was awakened way too early in the morning. Sleep was her only escape from her surroundings and it was ruined every day without fail. At around six thirty, the head resident, Dr. Mannon, with her deep red hair, would come to check on her. And every day it was the same questions ... any contractions? Any more bleeding? Any fluid leaking? Any fever? Anything different at all? It was a routine she knew like the back of her hand, and the answer was always, "Nothing's changed, and I'm still here."

Oh, another question that was asked every time when the attending physician would check on her was, "Can we do anything for you? There was an answer she gave without blinking an eye every single time, "Send me home." They could see how

114   andrea merkord

hard it was on her to be stuck there by herself, but there was nothing they could do about it. She was just too unstable to travel long distances.

### ISAIAH 38:17 NIV

Surely it was for my benefit that I suffered such anguish.
In your love you kept me from the pit of destruction.

On Thursday, September 5, she was given a tour of the NICU, or neonatal intensive care unit. They wanted to prepare her for the very likely chance that her baby could have an extended stay there and face great difficulties along the way. She was taken in a wheelchair down the hall and around the corner. This NICU was very large. They dealt with the sickest highest risk babies there are. They were able to show her a little girl who was at the same age that Thomas was that week. She was very tiny and all skin and bones.

The hospital social worker who had taken her down there also gave her a book to read about premature babies and the possible illnesses they faced and the machines they could be on at different stages of growth. She read it in no time and memorized it, just as she had done with all of the information they had received throughout their baby's complicated life.

Later that morning, Dr. Mannon came in and very carefully asked, "So, how was the NICU tour?"

Andrea just answered in a matter-of-fact way, "Fine."

"Were you surprised by anything? Did any of it scare you?"

"No, it was pretty much what I expected."

The doctor seemed surprised to hear that, as if she had expected to deal with some hysterical, shocked mother who didn't know what she was facing. Andrea kept surprising them in the way she made sure she was educated on every detail,

expect a miracle *115*

gruesome or not, about conditions and procedures they were dealing with. Education was the best way to control her fear. Her imagination was much worse than reality any day. It had always been the unknown that bothered her most.

Saturday, Andrea had to have another IV placement and blood drawn. As amazing as it sounds, yes, they had to do it twice again! Nothing feels better than a large IV needle missing its mark. That made eight different holes in her arms, not including any blood draws. Some were leaving permanent scars. She figured out, after trying different locations, that the ones in her arms were much better than a line in her hand. It just felt wrong in her hand, and she could always feel it whenever she ate, wrote, or switched the TV channel.

Amber called on Sunday, and they had only been on the phone for a few minutes when Andrea totally broke down and cried so heavily she could hardly speak. She just felt so lonely and scared. Amber felt far away and horrible that there was nothing she could do to help her sister. She couldn't control her own tears when she hung up the phone herself.

Immediately after that, Andrea called Sean and cried with him. During her down times, he was the one to raise her spirits.

"This is what we have to do right now. I don't know why this is happening to us, but we both believe that there is a reason for everything, right? We have to stay strong. God left you there for a reason. Maybe that's where you're getting the best care. You have to think of it that way, okay?"

Sean was her perfect partner. He was up when she needed him to be, and she returned the favor on his low days. When he would complain about how life is so unfair, they didn't deserve it, she would say, "Life isn't fair. What made you think it's an even playing field? You can't say that you want other people to go through this, too, to make it fair. I wouldn't wish this on anyone. God will never give you more than you can bear. The Bible promises that, and we both believe it, right? I don't know what the ultimate plan is, and from where I'm sitting, it seems a little ridiculous to go through all of this to have a baby, but that's why we're not the ones in charge. We left our chances to God, and we need to trust Him with the decisions. Sometimes the answer to the question is no, and we need to be prepared for that possibility."

They had perfect timing in being the opposite of each other. On only a couple of occasions were they both depressed at the same time, and then, they could cry together. That's okay, too, sometimes.

When Dr. Sandberg wasn't there, the perinatologist who checked on her was usually Dr. Ball. He was thin with very dark, somewhat spiky hair, and usually wore a sleeveless vest over his scrubs. *It sets him apart from other people*, she thought. He seemed genuinely concerned for her comfort and on Monday, September 9, day nineteen, he got her off the twenty-four hour monitoring.

He explained to her that things had been stable, but there was a small risk that being off of the monitor they could miss something substantial. She understood that it was a low risk, but he had to explain it anyway. She felt free. It was amazing to be able to sleep and get comfortable in any position she wanted without worrying that Thomas's heart rate got lost again. She could get up to go to the bathroom without carrying the cords around with her and plugging back in as soon as she was back in bed.

The new deal was this: She would be monitored twice each day, once at the beginning of the day shift and once at the beginning of the evening shift. Each shift was seven to seven. Usually, she would just get the straps out and hook herself up long before her new nurse came in to introduce herself. Andrea

expect a miracle *117*

was the easiest patient; she was usually the last patient they would check on at night. Many times they would come in and say, "Well, let's do your non-stress test now."

Andrea would show them the screen, and she had already hooked herself up for about half an hour and unhooked herself again. They had a long strip of the baby's heart rate to look at and it was all done.

It felt good to be in control of something again. That small, but substantial change gave Andrea a new view. When she spoke with Sean that evening, she was almost ready to accept her circumstances and deal with the fact that she was there for the long haul. That was a huge step for her, and maybe the place God had wanted her heart to be, before offering her the chance to go home.

### PSALM 46:10 NIV
#### Be still, and know that I am God;

On Tuesday, Dr. Ball shocked her by mentioning getting her to Portland, Oregon. Every Tuesday, the staff physicians at the hospital had a meeting to discuss things such as individual patient care. He told her that he would mention the possibility of transferring her to a Portland hospital, preferably Emanuel, since they were familiar with her case, or even St. Charles in Bend. Emanuel was more likely since she was still at a very volatile stage and they were the higher-rated hospital for mother and baby care.

She called Sean at nine o'clock on the dot, as she did every evening. Usually, she sat there with the phone on the rolling meal tray in front of her for about five minutes before it was time to call. She often had a game of solitaire going on the tiny table while she watched TV. Sean's sister, Karla, had sent her a package with just the kind of stuff she needed to keep herself entertained. A deck of playing cards, a hand held *Simon* game, about a dozen magazines to read, and best of all . . . nail polish and remover. She painted her toenails and finger nails about every other day. It was all she had to feel the slightest bit feminine in her hospital gown day in and day out. Each morning she wondered, *Hmm, what should I wear today; a hospital gown, or maybe, oh, a hospital gown? Good choice.*

She had quite the routine going to get through the days though. At about six thirty, she was awakened by a resident who asked her the same questions again and again. "Any more bleeding? Any contractions? Any concerns?" Then they would feel her legs and ask if they hurt because of lack of use. She was supposed to be bedridden, but she didn't stay "in bed" all day.

"Has anything changed?"

"No."

The same responses each and every morning. She would attempt to go back to sleep without much luck. At seven, she would watch *Little House on the Prairie,* her favorite childhood program. She owned most of the episodes on video at home. At about seven thirty, breakfast was served. The same lady usually delivered her meals throughout the week. She probably wondered if Andrea was ever going to leave that room.

At nine the excitement really began with *Live, With Regis and Kelly.* Everyone who stays home sick from school or work knows what's on at ten, right? *The Price Is Right,* of course. There was nothing on at eleven, so that was when she planned to take her showers. She treasured those moments out of bed daily and made them last as long as possible. She eventually ran out of the shampoo and conditioner she had brought and kept needing to ask the nurses for more. They would bring some to her in small cups that would last a few days each. Then she would be asking for more, feeling dependant on other people again.

Twelve o'clock was *Magnum,* p.i., and more importantly,

expect a miracle *119*

lunch time. One o'clock was *Animal Planet's Emergency Vets.* Not much was on TV after that, so either she read a book or magazine or played cards with the funnest person, of course, herself. Sometimes she would try to take an afternoon nap, but for some reason it made her feel guilty to do so. She already felt useless where she was and didn't want to be lazy as well, whatever that meant. As if watching TV or reading a magazine were any more productive than sleep was. Anywho, back to the daily schedule, from which one cannot deviate.

*Oprah* was on at four, followed by the news. Andrea hated watching the news at home because she felt it was too depressing, but there it was her only connection with the outside world. The evening was filled with the alternating evening programming that entertained most of America's households. Late at night, she could usually find a movie to watch. That was, of course, after calling Sean at nine. Whew, could it have been any more exciting? She had never watched so much television in her life, nor would she want to again.

The next time Dr. Ball came in, he told her there was no objection to sending her home after twenty-eight weeks. That would be the following Monday! They would take her off of the medications that were supposed to be keeping her contractions at bay, and if she remained stable, they could discuss taking a flight home.

While she was having her IV site changed for the umpteenth time, she pondered how she would get home to Oregon. Would she take a commercial flight? She still had the free flight from Alaska Airlines. It would only be a few hours away from medical help, but would that be too long? It was pretty risky to travel with bags and to do as much walking as would be required to travel through an airport, especially not knowing how her body would take movement after all that time. It was a lot to think about.

Sean was checking on airfare to come back down to visit Andrea, but the prices were astronomical and unreasonable. With all of the discussion going on about Andrea going back up to Oregon, Sean also wondered if he should just wait and see what happened with that first. Andrea tried to keep her journal up to date and continued doing quick little video clips every few days to update the viewing audience on her (lack of) progress.

At one point, Dr. Farmer stopped by Andrea's room and said, "You're still here?"

She had gone on vacation for two weeks and rubbed it in to poor little Andrea. Carol had also gone on vacation to visit her sister in New Mexico for a week. No matter what she was doing, she would manage to give Andrea a call every single night while she was gone. It was a thoughtful gesture. Andrea's own parents weren't calling very often. She just didn't understand why her parents didn't see how badly she needed them to be there for her.

Thursday, September 12, was day twenty-two. She had blood taken again, and nurses told her they had scheduled her for an MRI the following morning. She remembered back when they had returned home from the first surgery, the doctors wanted her to return later that month for a follow up MRI on Thomas's brain, but she didn't want to go back. Guess that problem was solved, wasn't it?

With the chance he could have suffered some kind of stroke or devastating situation in his brain caused by the first surgery, Andrea didn't really want to know what they could see. There was too much to deal with already and they never received good news, not once. She was also scared of being rolled into a tiny space where she couldn't move her arms. She figured they get some pretty big people in those things, so she shouldn't have too much difficulty.

expect a miracle    121

That made her feel better until seven o'clock on Friday morning came around. She was taken downstairs in a wheelchair and climbed onto a table that pulled her into the MRI machine. She was amazed at how tight the quarters actually were. If she bent her elbows at all, they touched the sides, which made her feel like stretching them out all the way, so she tried to keep them right at her sides so she wouldn't notice the closeness of them. With her eyes open, she could see the top of the tube just inches from her face. She wanted to pull back from it, which was impossible because she was lying on her back. She tried to keep her eyes closed during the scan so she wouldn't go crazy in there.

There were times when a man would come over the intercom and tell her when to hold her breath and let it out again. That at least gave her something to do to keep her mind busy. The entire scan only lasted about a half an hour. It wasn't too bad, she thought, once she reached minimum safe distance from it. It was a long day waiting to hear what the results were. There was no getting her mind off of it. She had no desire to know that information, but now that someone had the details, it was just eating at her to know the truth. After a long and difficult day of waiting, Dr. Sandberg came in and told her all looked fine. It was an anti-climactic moment.

She almost couldn't believe her ears. *I'm sorry, this is where you're supposed to say something horrible for me to ponder for the next week of my life*, she thought.

When she called Sean, he breathed a deep sigh of relief also. It just wasn't normal to get great news. What a nice change! And the most ironic part of the day, it was Friday the 13th.

**PROVERBS 15:30 NIV**

A cheerful look brings joy to the heart, and
good news gives health to the bones.

# GARDETTOS, ANYONE?

**JEREMIAH 32:27 NIV**
I am the Lord, the God of all mankind. Is anything too hard for me?

After surviving Friday the 13th, and ironically receiving their first piece of good news on that day, Andrea started considering what it would be like to travel home in her condition. She thought about how long it would take to get through each step. From the cab ride, checking in bags, flight time, baggage claim, and getting a ride to Emanuel Hospital in Portland, it would only be a few hours away from medical care. The more she thought about those *few hours,* the more it seemed like a risky time period. Even if she had a wheelchair through the airports, it would be a lot more activity than she had been used to for more than three weeks. With her water broken, even if she remained stable, the cord could prolapse and cut off Thomas's oxygen supply and she would be helpless to do anything about it. Her imagination got carried away, and she pictured herself on a plane at thirty thousand feet and feeling something very wrong happening with a rush of emergent activity while her baby died inside of her. She felt like the worst mother in the world. If there was even the slightest chance of that happening, how could she live with herself for putting him at risk after all they'd been through already?

Her desire to find a way back to Oregon was unchallenged, but her eagerness for travel the next week had dropped to a new low. On Saturday morning, Sean called her bright and

expect a miracle

early from his dad's house. They were both bachelors that week and decided to keep each other company.

Sean asked her, "What would you think if we went to the casino today?"

"No. I don't think that's a good idea. I'm not bringing in any money and our bills are going to be astronomical when I get out of here, not to mention Thomas's bills, since he's going to spend some time in the hospital too," Andrea said.

At that, Sean got upset and blurted out the reasons he thought it would be just fine and how he needed to get away and just have some fun for a day.

"Well, so would I! I don't get to escape, do I? This is happening inside my body, remember? I couldn't escape from it if I wanted to. Sometimes I wish I could just forget about it for only a minute, but that's impossible. I don't want you to go. Be responsible this time."

They hung up the phone on bad terms. Andrea broke down crying. She never liked arguing with Sean, and, truth be told, they didn't have conflict very often. She was crushed that he was so far away and they couldn't be together to make them both feel better. As she was attempting to wipe away her tears before anyone saw her, Dr. Sandberg came in the room. He could see she was upset. Her eyes were red. He asked her if something was wrong.

"I just had a bad phone conversation, that's all," she answered.

"With your husband?" the doctor asked.

"Yeah," and a long pause. She went on to explain what they had argued over.

"We like to go to the casino every once in a while and just have fun with a preset amount of money, but that was when we had money to blow. We have a different situation now. We need to prepare for our new medical bills that are piling up as

124  andrea merkord

we speak. I always end up playing the bad guy. I hate it, but I'm not going to back down."

No sooner had he left the room, Andrea picked up the phone and apologized about the argument and caved in.

"I want you to have a good day, and I hate fighting with you like this. We don't need to be arguing about stupid things. Okay?"

Sean was excited about going and made sure to call her a couple of times while he was there. There were some slot machines that they both enjoyed playing. In certain situations, the computer takes players to a bonus round where they get to choose their prize. When Sean got to one of those bonus rounds, he called Andrea and asked her which parrot to choose. She told him to choose the blue one for Thomas. Unfortunately, she didn't get to find out what the prize was because a casino staff person told him he couldn't use a cell phone in there. They quickly said their good-byes.

Not long after talking with Sean, Andrea's nurse came in to change her IV site again. She had kept track of how many IV needles had been in her arms, and that one made ten different locations. People had always told her, "When you're pregnant, you'll get so used to needles that it won't bother you anymore."

Bologna! She had had more needles in her arms than she would have ever expected, and she would never get used to it. She couldn't see the light at the end of the tunnel. She hadn't even needed the IV line for about a week but was required to leave it in "just in case."

On Sunday, September 15, a.k.a. *Day twenty-five*, the nurse asked her if she had been weighed recently.

"No, I don't think I've been weighed at all. I'd be curious to know how huge I am," she said.

**expect a miracle** *125*

"Well, I'll bring in the scale later today and we'll find out. How's that sound?"

Andrea thought, *It's pretty bad when all you have to get excited about is getting weighed.* The nurse eventually wheeled in a large and cumbersome scale on wheels. She took a moment to plug it in and reset it. Andrea could not believe what she saw when she stepped up onto it. She had gained a whopping ... one and a half pounds. She had gained only a pound and a half in twenty-eight weeks of pregnancy. She knew she had been losing muscle with all of the time spent in bed, but it was actually much worse than she thought.

## 2 CORINTHIANS 12:9 NIV

But he said to me, "My grace is sufficient for you, for my power is made perfect in weakness." Therefore I will boast all the more gladly about my weaknesses, so that Christ's power may rest on me.

The big day finally arrived, twenty-eight weeks, that magical marker in pregnancy when you jump into a much safer category for preemies born at that age. It was a great relief and very exciting because it also meant that the doctors would start discussing travel plans for a possible trip to Oregon. The *plan* was to take her off of the Nifedepine and see how she did. If she remained stable, Dr. Ball had told her she could make plans to travel.

At ten thirty Monday morning, she had an ultrasound downstairs. Thomas was continuing to gain weight and everything else looked fine, except for the obvious missing fluid. Thomas didn't have any room to move around in there, which was also another disappointing part of the pregnancy to Andrea. She was missing out on all of the fun movement other moms got to experience. What else could be taken away from her? The more she thought about all of the things she had originally been looking forward to, the bitterer she became about how unfair it was.

Dr. Sandberg came by her room later and told her that he would discuss her condition in the Tuesday staff meeting the next day and see if travel was a feasible option. Again, that made her feel excited, but anxious. She could really be going home, she thought, or at least back to Oregon. To Oregonians, it is considered a privilege to live there. It's a beautiful state to live in, and it seems like everyone who moves there comes out of California. Andrea herself was born in Anaheim, California, and Sean was born in New Mexico. Both of them had spent almost all of their lives living in Oregon, and they badly wanted Thomas to be a true Oregonian.

On Tuesday afternoon, Dr. Sandberg came back in and sat down in the chair at the foot of Andrea's bed. In the meeting they had decided that a commercial flight was a bad idea. The best way would be to try to arrange some kind of medical transport. He told her they would have someone call her insurance to begin some preparations if possible. Andrea didn't know quite how to feel. She was somewhat disappointed but hopeful transport could be arranged. The only question she had was how long would that take to arrange? She was feeling down that afternoon and even though her nurse had brought in new sheets for the bed and a new gown, she never got out of bed to take the shower she usually looked so forward to.

A tall Asian lady named Karen came in later to let Andrea know what the insurance said. Her policy covered six thousand dollars per year for any kind of emergency transport. The early figures on her trip added up to over nine thousand dollars. Andrea thought about whether it would be worth the trip if they had to fork out three thousand dollars of their own money. That was a huge expense.

Just a short while later, Karen came back and gave her

expect a miracle *127*

more news. For Andrea's safety, they would need to use the larger jet, which would total twelve thousand dollars! Andrea could hardly believe her ears. She thought to herself, *Twelve thousand dollars to get from San Francisco to Portland. Unbelievable. Is that going via France?* She knew there was no way they could justify the extra expense. Karen did shine a small amount of light on it. There was a chance they could get the insurance to cover the entire cost of transport to save themselves money in the long run. It made a lot of sense for the insurance to pay for the transport because of how much it was costing them every day to keep Andrea in a high-risk hospital like UCSF. It would be less expensive in the long run to have her in Portland. There was still a shred of hope. That's all Andrea needed to keep going.

Christina continued to call Andrea every day, usually in the morning. It was wonderful that she made such an effort to provide Andrea with words of encouragement and a way to pass some time each day. On Wednesday morning, Andrea decided that after she was finished doing her own "non stress test" again, she would just hop in the shower without calling the nurse. She still had the linens from the day before when she skipped her shower and made her own bed after getting out of the bathroom. It was gratifying to do a little bit of taking care of herself. Just to do something simple like making her own bed made her feel more at home. Later, when her nurse asked if she would like to take her shower so she could change the sheets, Andrea confessed to what she had been up to.

"You are the easiest patient I've ever had." The nurse could only laugh.

They had decided to put Andrea back on the monitor for a while because she had a lot of contracting, and Thomas's heart rate was dipping low quite a bit. While she lay on her side, it was hard to concentrate on anything but the monitor. Those times were always stressful. With each contraction she would hold her breath and wait for Thomas's heart rate to climb back up to a safe level. She knew what to look for on the monitor, and she knew what was safe and what was dangerous. For the rest of the day she remained on the monitor.

Dr. Mannon knew how down Andrea had felt and always tried to make her feel better. She knew Andrea had no personal effects with her and no pictures of home, so she brought in a picture of her own cat to brighten the room a little bit. The animal in the photo suited the doctor. They were both red heads. It was a very kind gesture and much appreciated by Andrea, though she never let Dr. Mannon know how much. For some reason, she still had her guard up.

She had mentioned to Dr. Mannon how much she missed having Subway sandwiches, and she remembered there was one across the street that Sean and Tony had gone to when they were there. She was somewhat surprised when Dr. Mannon told her it was okay for her to go over there and pick up some food if she wanted to. Andrea got dressed in her own clothes and did her hair and make-up for the first time in days. She made sure to wear a long-sleeved shirt to cover up the IV just above her left wrist. The doctor joked that it might freak out the person making her food if they saw the huge IV. She also told Andrea to take her time and enjoy walking around, but they would put her on the monitor when she returned to double check that everything was fine. That sounded like a fair trade off to Andrea.

After twenty-nine days, Andrea was finally walking out of the maternity ward on her own two feet. That was the last time she would walk out on her own. To any other person she passed, she was just another lady, not a local maternity ward resident. It was dignifying to carry her purse down the hall and get on the elevator. It actually made her a little dizzy going all the way down to the first floor. When she stepped outside, it was an indescribable feeling of freedom. Just a taste of normal life. Like any other day at work when she would run down to get herself a sandwich and eat it at her desk. Her friends at work poked fun at her saying, "Thomas is going to come out addicted to Dr. Pepper and Subway sandwiches."

For the first time in a month, she enjoyed ordering her favorite (and only) sandwich. Why ruin a good thing by trying something new? Remember? A six-inch Subway Melt on wheat with American cheese, plenty of lettuce, little onion, tomatoes, extra mayonnaise, olives, and extra salt and pepper. Simple, but perfect to her. Manna from heaven! The smell of the sandwich shop hovered in her nostrils. She always thought it would be great to have a Subway-scented candle in her kitchen. She couldn't wait to get it back and sink her teeth into it. But, before heading back to the confines of her room too soon, she went to an adjacent bookstore and picked up a spiral notebook for writing letters or just keeping notes. She also looked around the gift shop before stepping back onto the elevator and heading back to the fifteenth floor.

She tried to enjoy the long walk down the halls and her last few moments of freedom. Dr. Mannon smiled at her when she got closer to her room, directly across from the nurses' station. It was probably strange to see Andrea as a normal person for once and what she would look like under better circumstances. Maybe another time and another place.

Before eating her sandwich, she wrapped her belly with the straps she so dreaded and began her testing to make sure things didn't get too worked up on her travels. Thomas looked and sounded great on the monitor as Andrea enjoyed her lunch.

## MATTHEW 7:7 NIV

Ask and it will be given to you; seek and you will find;
knock and the door will be opened to you.

When she got her IV out and didn't have to get another in its place, Andrea knew things were looking up. *They must be preparing for transport,* she thought. It was Friday and three days since they had started discussing things with her insurance. There was a lot of negotiating going on, and Karen was great about letting Andrea know when anything new came about. They were having a lot of forms faxed to them. She just thought, *Well, at least that's not a 'No' yet.*

She would have to wait for Monday before any kind of arrangements could be made. Dr. Ball told her he was pretty sure nothing would happen over the weekend, so she settled in for another weekend in her tiny room. On Saturday, though, she had a visitor, her Aunt Janie, her mother's sister who lived about an hour and a half from San Francisco. They hadn't seen each other in many years, and it was nice to have a visit. Janie called her before leaving home and asked her if there was anything she needed.

Andrea thought for a second and said, "You're gonna laugh, but I just ran out of deodorant."

"What kind do you use?" Janie asked.

"Secret, Powder Fresh."

Janie said, "You're not going to believe this, but I have a brand new one right here in my cupboard. I bought a double pack."

"You're right, I don't believe it. That's great."

Andrea laughed inside at how strange it was to talk about deodorant with someone she hadn't seen since middle school.

"Is there anything else I can bring?"

expect a miracle *131*

Andrea thought again, "Well, if it's not too much to ask, is there a Christian bookstore on your way?"

Janie said, "Yes, there's one near here."

"Do you know the *Left Behind* series of books? I haven't read the latest one yet. Sean tried to get it for me before he left but couldn't find it."

"No problem. I'll see if I can get one for you. All right then, I should be there in a couple of hours." Janie hung up.

That was another day Andrea had an excuse to do her hair and make-up. She took her time, as usual, in the shower and was anticipating her first visitor since Sean left twenty days earlier. Not only that, but an aunt she hadn't seen for a very long time.

When Janie arrived, no one would have placed her as Andrea's relative. Her large six-foot stature was the exact opposite of Andrea's petite one. (They never could figure out what gene pool Andrea came from that made her so short). Andrea got out of bed to give her a hug and Janie was nervous about her getting up from bed rest and said, "No, no, no, stay in bed."

She brought her a very large basket full of baby gifts for Thomas, which included some preemie-sized clothing and bottles, and she brought the deodorant and the book Andrea had requested.

They had a nice visit during which she gave Janie the run down of the events that led them to their current predicament. Janie told her what she had been up to since her third husband of nearly twenty years had died suddenly of a heart attack just a couple of years before. She seemed to be well and Andrea was glad. Janie hadn't had it easy in many times of her life and she wished her the best. After a couple of hours, Janie hit the road and headed back home.

Throughout the afternoon, Thomas's heart rate kept dropping and it concerned Dr. Mannon to the point that she made Andrea remain on the baby monitors throughout the night. Andrea wasn't as annoyed by the monitor as she previously had been when she was on them twenty-four hours a day with no relief. That time she was worried about Thomas and not having Sean there to make her feel better. When they had their nightly conversation, she was sure to tell him that Thomas had been having trouble. The last thing she wanted to do was worry him, but not keeping him informed left him out of the important details he was missing out on being so far away.

Sunday, Andrea was surprised when Dr. Mannon told her it was her last day as Chief Resident on that ward. She was moving on to another hospital not too far away. She made a point to come and tell Andrea that news, and there was a moment of silence when Andrea should have said more but didn't. She had been well taken care of, and the doctor had made a conscious effort to make her feel at home as best she could. With that, she walked out of Andrea's life forever. Later, Andrea would deeply regret keeping her thoughts to herself and not opening up to her.

PSALM 116:6 NIV

The Lord protects the simple hearted; when
I was in great need, he saved me.

The new chief began the next day by introducing himself to Andrea and quickly learned she wasn't a happy camper. She gave him the cold shoulder and gave the briefest answers she could to his questions to get him out of the room. She should have just stopped them every morning and said, "Okay, let's go down the checklist . . . the bleeding's the same, the fluid's the same, no, there's no pain in my legs, everything's the same, and *no, I don't have any questions.*" Her bitterness was obvious and

expect a miracle *133*

she made no attempt to conceal it. She just wanted to survive one day at a time.

On his second day of checking on Andrea and getting heavy sighs when he turned the light on at six o'clock AM, he said, "I'm sorry about waking you, but we have to ask you these questions."

She answered them again and tried her best to go back to sleep before the food service came in at seven. After breakfast, Dr. Ball came in and she was glad to see him. She always saved her questions for the specialists. Either Dr. Sandberg or Dr. Ball were her chosen ones. She trusted them.

Dr. Ball told her, "I'm going to try to get to the bottom of the insurance deal this week for you. I'll do my best."

She just smiled back and said, "Alrighty then."

There was no news on Tuesday, which was already a week since they had begun discussions with the insurance company about payment. On Wednesday, Andrea's spirits were soon to be lifted higher than they had been in thirty days.

Karen came in and blurted out, "They approved your transport. One hundred percent paid. They are faxing the approval this morning and we should be getting you out of here this afternoon."

The first thing Andrea did was call Sean at work. He couldn't believe his ears.

"They did?" he asked.

She was almost in tears and said, "That means I get to see you soon. I'm so excited I can hardly contain myself. The people around here won't recognize me if I'm happy."

Sean had to get back to work, "That's great news, honey. I'm happy for you too. I love you."

"I love you too," she said and hung up.

She immediately got up to take her shower. Since her IV had been taken out, she didn't have to wrap her arm anymore to protect it, which was much easier. She had gone five days without that darn iv and it felt wonderful. She experienced such a rush of excitement that after her shower and curling her hair, putting make-up on, and putting her own clothes on, she started getting her things in order. Her rush of energy didn't stop until almost lunch time. She piled up all of her magazines so other patients could read them. The stereo she had been using was placed on the wide window sill right beside them. She carefully packed up the video camera after making a last scan of her room, the place she had been confined to for more than a month. She ended the video in front of the mirror, smile plastered to her cheeks, telling everyone watching that she was on her way home, or at least to Portland, Oregon, which was good enough for her.

With her belongings in a neat pile and her suitcase packed, she moved her bed away from the window and back to its original location near the center of the room. She tried to remember where everything had been before Sean left. He had reorganized her space for her so everything would be within arm's reach. She knew if she got caught moving the bed or computer stand, she would be killed by her doctors, but no one caught her in the act or asked about her room being remodeled that day.

Throughout her time on the fifteenth floor, she had ventured out more and more from her room. She started going down to the family waiting rooms to check out what was in the vending machines at the end of the hall. One afternoon she was in bed eating a package of Gardettos that really hit the spot. She got to the crumbs at the bottom of the bag and poured out the remaining small chunks into her left hand. Thinking there wasn't much left, she opened up wide and popped them into her mouth in one swift motion. She immediately realized there was more left in the bag than there had originally seemed, and

expect a miracle *135*

her small mouth was stuffed too full to chew comfortably. She was in that uncomfortable state at precisely the moment Dr. Ball knocked on the door and came into the room. She didn't know what to do when he said, "Hello." All she could do was try to chew the snack in her mouth while her face turned beat red. The doctor quietly waited for her to be done making a pig of herself. As she chewed the rest of her crunchy snack, she thought to herself, "Oh my gosh! He probably thinks that's what I do all day in here is just stuff my face like a disgusting pig." It topped her list as one of the most embarrassing moments of her life.

Dr. Ball needed her to sign some paperwork before she left. He told her, "Read it carefully before you sign it."

It read in part . . .

> The patient is very interested in back transport to Portland, Oregon, and continued inpatient care at Emanuel Hospital there under the care of Maternal-fetal medicine. She understands that transport may be associated with risks to her and the fetus, with poor outcome being likely if she delivers en route or has significant hemorrhage . . . She understands that the clinical situation remains tenuous and that she remains at risk for pre-term labor and delivery as well as fetal compromise and even stillbirth . . . With full understanding of these risks she wishes to proceed.

After signing that, she felt like the worst mother in the world again. What was wrong with her?

Karen stopped by her room after lunch and told her that she was under the impression that her ride would be there in the late afternoon, maybe around five o'clock or so. She could see the giddiness in Andrea's eyes and had an idea of how thrilling that must have been for her. The afternoon was dragging on as she stood by the window thinking, *This is the last time I'll be staring at the Golden Gate Bridge, and at the football field across the block, and at the little street where our San Francisco journey began, and at all of the joggers I've been so jealous of throughout the sunny days of September, my favorite month in Bend, which I've almost completely missed.*

### JAMES 1:2–4 NIV

Consider it pure joy, my brothers, whenever you face trials of many kinds, because you know that the testing of your faith develops perseverance. Perseverance must finish its work so that you may be mature and complete, not lacking anything.

At nearly five o'clock, Karen came back in and explained why there was a delay.

"What's happening is you're basically hitching a ride on someone else's transport while they're in our area. That patient being moved is waiting for a bed to open up at the location he's being moved to. Apparently, they don't know when that will be. I'm sorry, there won't be any transport happening tonight."

With her extreme happiness crushed to oblivion, Andrea shouldn't have been surprised by the news she had received. Nothing had gone right up to that point, why should the transport be any different? Her bitterness was back with full force when she picked up the phone to call Sean.

She began, "Guess where I am? Portland, you ask? No! That would mean something actually went right for once, but this is us we're talking about, remember? Nothing works out the way we think it should."

Sean asked with confusion and disappointment in his tone, "What happened? Why haven't you left?"

expect a miracle *137*

Through her flood of tears, she said, "They never came to get me."

He could hear the sounds of her crushed spirit and started to cry himself. She explained that they were waiting for someone else's ride to happen because her insurance wouldn't pay for it any other way.

"So it sounds like you should be coming tomorrow. Don't cry, honey. You'll be here soon."

He tried to raise her hopes a little, even thought he knew she would be spending another night in that same room. They had been sent on another roller coaster ride of pure joy followed by sudden overwhelming disappointment. Sean kept asking God why life wasn't fair.

"Why is this happening to us? Why doesn't every couple have to go through this to have a baby? And we still aren't guaranteed a healthy outcome! Why?" His frustration was building at home, though he did his best to hide it from Andrea.

Thursday, day thirty-six, came and went. Followed by Friday, then Saturday and Sunday. Dr. Sandberg came in to check on Andrea and see how she was holding up after such a shocking turn of events.

Andrea told him, "Well, after this, you're gonna need to go ahead and transfer me to the psych ward, cause that's where I'm headed!"

She saw the doctor laugh for the first time since she had been there.

On Monday morning, when Dr. Ball came in the room, he seemed to be the only person around who understood her heartache. He was the only one she smiled at. He appeared to be frustrated himself at the delay of the transport. He wanted her to go while she was still stable. He promised her he would get to the bottom of it one way or another.

Tuesday, October 1, came in with the usual fog hovering

over the bay like plastic wrap. Andrea couldn't see anything below the tenth floor windows. It appeared to be a bright, crisp day outside though. She thought out loud, "Well, I missed the entire month of September at home. It's such a beautiful month in Bend. I can't believe I've been sitting here since August 22. Holy cow! That's a long time."

Her monologue continued internally,

*If I had known from the beginning I would be here for this long, I don't think I could have come out of it with my sanity. At least I hung onto little shreds of hope along each step of the way, thinking I would be going home, only to be disappointed repeatedly. I really don't know which is worse, having all of our bad news at once or continuing repeated assaults to the mind and soul with one piece of heartbreaking news after another. We weren't given a choice of how to face this ordeal. We just take what keeps coming our way with faith and hope that it will all turn out alright in the end. The question is, when will that end come?*

She was deep in thought and gazing out the window when there was a knock on the door.

"Andrea, it's Karen. I have great news. The transport has been arranged for today."

Without much enthusiasm, Andrea responded with, "Yeah, okay."

Karen continued, "They're picking you up after they are finished transporting another patient to San Diego or something. It will be late afternoon and they will call when they are getting closer. I'll keep you informed." She closed the door behind her on the way out.

Only a few short minutes later, Dr. Ball came into the room.

"I heard they are supposed to come get you today finally. How are you doing?"

She said, "Everything's the same. Just waiting here as I

expect a miracle *139*

have been since last Wednesday. I just want to get closer to home. I want to see my husband."

Dr. Ball shook her hand and told her, "I hope I *don't* see you in here tomorrow."

Andrea picked up the phone and called Sean at his work number.

"Well, yet again, they are supposed to come pick me up this afternoon. I don't know whether to jump for joy now or not. Anyway, I'll let you know if anything actually transpires today. Love you."

That time she made no extra effort to get herself worked up about leaving that tiny room. She did take her shower and took the time to look decent. What could it hurt, right? For the last time she made herself a comfy spot in her hospital bed to sit and pass the afternoon with the television and her solitaire games. She made another video of herself in the room and had to correct her last video entry.

"Well, " she said, "I lied. I didn't get to leave when I last taped myself and told you I was going to Portland. Today is Tuesday, October 1, day forty-one, and I'm rescheduled to be transported today. I'll let ya know if that really happens," she said with a hint of sarcasm as she turned off the camera just before lunch arrived.

Inside she was nervous and excited, although she tried to repress those feelings. She didn't want to be crushed again if bad news came instead of her flight home. Five o'clock came, then five thirty. Finally, at nearly six o'clock, there was a knock at her door. It was her nurse with Karen. Her transport had arrived. She was actually leaving that place.

She was sitting in the chair in the corner of the room eating her dinner, a grilled ham and cheese sandwich and white rice, which she had ordered off the special request menu. She didn't like what they were serving for the regular dinner that night. Quickly, she ate her sandwich and grabbed her bags, which, for the most part, were still ready to go. She also had the basketful of gifts from Aunt Janie, which she didn't want to forget.

A masculine lady with long brown hair came into the room to grab her bags for her. She looked around the room slightly confused.

"Are you Andrea?"

"Yes, I've been waiting for you," Andrea said with a smile.

"Okay." She laughed. "I'm just not used to my patients walking around. Most of them are in bed. Let me get your stuff and we'll be ready for you."

Andrea paused to look out the window and around her room for the very last time. She was surprised to feel a sense of sadness at leaving that part of her life behind her. She was excited and uneasy to see what was in store for her next though. They hooked her up to portable monitors for blood pressure and what not and wheeled her out on the ambulance gurney. To her it was a tremendous moment to be celebrated, but as she left the maternity ward, life continued at a hurried pace, just as it had before her arrival forty-one days earlier.

### PSALM 116:7 NIV
Be at rest once more, O my soul, for the Lord has been good to you.

Andrea was experiencing total elation at the thought that she was actually going back to Oregon. Her ride was there and she was officially on her way. The transport personnel made their way down to the ambulance bay and packed Andrea's belongings wherever they could find a safe place. Her gurney was in a seated position for her, and she was placed in the ambulance facing the back doors. Everyone found their seatbelts and they

expect a miracle  *141*

were on their way to the airport. The driver told her it would be about a thirty-minute ride.

While her transport nurse was writing down her stats on a chart, Andrea took a peak at all of the equipment stored in such a tiny space. She began to feel sick to her stomach and asked, "Do you have any vomit bags, just in case?"

The nurse asked, "Are you feeling sick?"

Andrea said, "Well, I'm starting to. I've always gotten motion sickness and it's been worse since I've been pregnant. It's better to be safe than sorry."

They searched around for something to catch it just in case she did get sick, and she hung onto it throughout the ride. She could see out the two small back windows, one in each door. It was strange to be watching the driver in the lane behind them. She thought, *I wonder if they can see me in here looking at them.*

Suddenly, the urge came over her and she threw up before she could warn anybody else. She was embarrassed to be subjecting those other people to her problems in such a confined space. It sounded horrible and smelled worse. The nurse was very helpful and took it away for her.

At the airport, they entered through a private gate away from the main terminal. There was a Lear jet waiting there for them with two pilots finishing their dinner. Andrea was allowed to climb onto the plane herself and sit in a regular seat instead of remaining on the gurney for the entire flight. It was a small plane with seating for nine, including the pilots. Andrea kept thinking, *There's one more step behind me.* She wanted to be prepared for the slightest chance that her hopes would be smashed to bits again and something would keep her from making it to Portland that day. Everything was going fine so far. She could just see herself involved in a plane crash and ending up back at UCSF, right back where she started.

The ride was the smoothest one she had ever been on.

andrea merkord

Did that make it worth the twelve thousand dollar fare? She thought not. She and the nurse got into a brief conversation about Andrea's ordeal up to that point. As with most people she talked to, including medical professionals, the lady was shocked at the story and the continuing saga. Before she knew it, they had arrived at the Portland airport and another step of the trip was behind her. She thought, *There's no taking me back now! I've made it to Oregon.* She looked around the lights of the city she knew so well. Although she didn't live there, it was a great feeling of coming home again.

## 2 SAMUEL 22:29 NIV

You are my lamp, O Lord;
the Lord turns my darkness into light.

Andrea was placed on the gurney again for the ride to the hospital in another ambulance. These drivers were very friendly and talkative, asking the transport nurses all about their travels that day. It was almost nine o'clock and they still had a flight back to New Mexico that night to get home. They had worked late to get Andrea to Portland. She was very grateful for that effort. Before they arrived at Legacy Emanuel Hospital, Andrea felt sick again and blessed those poor nurses with another dose of her partially digested dinner. It felt awkward to be facing the back of a vehicle, especially after not being in one at all for over a month.

Andrea was given a wheelchair and was wheeled up to the labor and delivery ward. The nurses there were awaiting her arrival and had everything ready for her. They wore scrubs with patterns on them, as opposed to the staff of UCSF, who all wore plain blue scrubs. It made the atmosphere a little more upbeat. The first thing Andrea did was make a short telephone call to

expect a miracle *143*

Sean and was hoping not to wake him. It was about nine thirty, and all she said was, "I'm here. I'm at Emanuel."

Her nurse was fairly short with petite features and dark brown, bobbed hair. She immediately gave Andrea a gown, *yay*, and got her hooked up to the baby monitors. She was having a large number of contractions after such a busy evening. Plus, the fact that she was finally taken off the medication, Nifedepine, which may or may not have been holding back her contractions all of that time. The nurse wanted her to remain on the monitors until the attending physician was out of the O.R.

She said, "It's Dr. Weick tonight, and he takes a long time in a C-section."

About an hour later, he came in to see her.

"We've been waiting for you," he said.

The first question on Andrea's mind was, "How long do you allow women on bed rest to go before you deliver them. At UCSF, they told me they would let me go as far as thirty-four weeks and then they would deliver. How far do you go here?"

She had already given them the first glimpse of her eagerness to be done with that whole pregnancy thing.

Dr. Weick said, "No, we won't deliver until thirty-five weeks if you don't go into labor on your own."

She was so disappointed, but she knew she had to take the good with the bad. At least she was in Oregon, and on Friday, Sean would be there to visit her. It wasn't until midnight that she was moved to her permanent location for the next many weeks on the other half of the maternity ward. Her room was much smaller than the one she had been in before. It would take time to orient herself with her new surroundings. For the time being, what she needed was sleep, and that's exactly what she did.

## JAMES 1:17 NIV

Every good and perfect gift is from above, coming
down from the father of the heavenly lights, who
does not change like shifting shadows.

Wednesday, October 2, Andrea awoke to a bright, sunny morning in Portland, Oregon. That was something she had been wishing for since Sean left her alone five weeks before. Her favorite Portland doctor was attending that day, and Dr. Di Federico came in bright and early to check-up on her.

"Good morning," she said. "We've been waiting for you for about a week now."

"Believe me, I know. I've been waiting to get here for longer," Andrea said with a grin from ear to ear.

They discussed Andrea's continued care at the new hospital, and the doctor told her she would be having an ultrasound that morning so they could get a look at how things were doing inside the babies' little world. Before lunch, she was wheeled downstairs and looked around as she reoriented herself with that facility. She had already been down those halls a few times before. The ultrasound rooms were small, and that time it was a man who did the scan. He didn't talk much, but Andrea watched what he was doing and she could see he was retaking the measurements of the major body parts, like leg bones, arms, and head circumference. There was still a major shortage of fluid, no surprise to anyone.

Early that afternoon, Amber called to see if Andrea would like a visitor.

Andrea said, "Of course I would. Are you kidding me?"

Amber said, "I'll be off of work in a couple of hours and I'll be by there after I pick up Brayden from daycare."

"You can come into the emergency room entrance. My

expect a miracle  *145*

room looks over the emergency room parking lot. I'm on the second floor maternity ward."

Andrea had new reasons to get up and put make-up on after her shower. Not only did it make her feel better, but she was meeting new doctors and nurses and just wanted to look better in general. She was given a new hospital mug that had a straw attached to the lid for water, and she was having the nurses fill it every time they came to her room. She felt bad because at UCSF, she was getting her own drinks most of the time, and she went through a lot of water every day. She probably drank it out of boredom while she watched TV more than anything else. She asked her nurse where the ice was so she could refill her own cup, and it just happened to be directly across the hall from her room.

Andrea's room was less sterile than her previous room, with painted walls and paintings hanging on them. There were also shelves for personal belongings and flower vases. Above her head was a wood cabinet for more storage and there was a radio with speakers in the ceiling. On her left side was a nightstand with a drawer where she kept her wallet and her playing cards. The bed was angled in the corner, and up to her right was the ceiling mounted television and a VCR. On the ground below, near the foot of her bed, was another cabinet, on which she placed her suitcase. Inside that cabinet was a mini fridge/freezer. She also faced the main room door and right next to that was the bathroom door.

The bathroom was much smaller than the last one with just a standing shower with a wooden bench that folded down from the tile for a seat. There was a small countertop where she placed her bathroom supplies. On the other side of her bed was a tall corner cabinet and a bed for a spouse. Underneath were a couple of drawers for blankets and other storage, and it laid directly below the windows, which faced out to the parking lot. She didn't mind the parking lot view, though, because she sat there watching squirrels run between the trees and bushes while dodging the people coming to and fro.

When Amber arrived with Brayden, they brought some flowers, which brightened up the room. They had a nice visit. It was wonderful for Andrea to see someone she loved. The next day was a work day for Amber, so she had to leave fairly early. Andrea was just glad someone had come to see her. She could hardly wait for Friday so she could see Sean. At nine o'clock, she made her usual call to Sean and told him all about her new surroundings and the visitor she had that day. They both welcomed the long-awaited changes.

Andrea spent a lot of the day Thursday learning the new TV channel choices, which weren't many. At UCSF, she had forty-one channels to choose from. At Emanuel, she had less than a dozen local channels. She had her daily routine of shows to watch that passed the time for her, but here she couldn't watch *Little House On The Prairie* in the morning; she didn't have that channel anymore. *Regis and Kelli* was on an hour later than she was used to. She didn't understand that because she was in the same time zone, just farther north. This interrupted *The Price Is Right* at ten o'clock. What was a girl to do? There was no *Animal Planet* to watch after lunch. Instead, it was the *Jenny Jones Show* or nothing at all. Most of the time she would choose nothing at all over shows like that one.

She still spent large amounts of time playing solitaire with the cards Karla had sent her or reading the book Aunt Janie brought to her. She was about halfway through the book by then. Andrea was never one to spend lengthy periods of time reading, because it always made her feel tired, and then she just felt like taking a nap. A nap, however, was the last thing on her mind on Friday, October 4. That was the day she had waited for since September 1. Sean was coming to spend the weekend

expect a miracle *147*

in her room with her. She felt like she was getting ready for a date. The excitement was pouring from her face all throughout the day.

Early in the morning, her sister-in-law, Tandi, called to verify the directions to the hospital from Eastern Oregon and to see if there was anything she could bring. They discussed a list of movies and books she would pack up with her. Tandi also whispered that she would steal some of Craig's Dr. Pepper. Craig was Sean's older brother by seven years, and the four of them spent many years enjoying each other's company. From camping trips with their Waverunners to Super Bowl Sundays, it was always a good time with lots of laughter. Sean and Tandi were the Pepsi drinkers of the group and Craig and Andrea were Dr. Pepper fans, so when Craig spotted Tandi walking out to the car with a six-pack of Dr. Pepper, he stopped her.

"Where are you taking my Dr. Pepper?" he asked.

"To your sister-in-law who's all by herself in Portland, unless you want me to tell her you wouldn't share with her," Tandi responded with a little teasing in her tone.

Tandi was on her way up to Washington to spend the week at Karla's watching Jordyn and Taylor while Karla left on a business trip for a week. Martin would be home, too, but Tandi would be filling in during the week since Karla usually stayed with the children and worked in the evenings doing home decorating shows. Portland was right on her way up to Washington, and it was a perfect chance to see the mysterious pregnant woman. Everyone knew she was pregnant but never got to see her that way! Andrea was accused of hoaxing everyone just to get some vacation time. That was not the type of vacation she would have chosen.

Andrea was glad to have another visitor. Life was getting more exciting every day. Wasn't she the popular one? Tandi brought some homemade cookies, which she knew Andrea loved. She also put the Dr. Pepper in the mini fridge for Andrea's enjoyment later. Andrea could hardly wait to drink them all. Tandi also brought a bunch of movies and some great inspirational books to read. Their visit was also a short one. Tandi had a long way to go, but it did give her a chance to stretch her legs a bit.

Now Andrea had nothing to do but wait. It was still hours before Sean would be coming and the time went by at a snail's pace. She would go sit in the window and watch the cars go in and out, counting the parking spaces that were available at any given moment. At some times, the parking lot would be full, and she would think, *Don't come now, Sean, there are no spaces open for you.*

Then cars would leave one, two, three at a time, and she would turn back to her TV to pass some more time. She couldn't believe the feeling of butterflies in her stomach. He was her own husband for Pete's sake, not some blind date. That's what made it perfect though. The man of her dreams was on his way to see the woman of his own dreams and their first baby boy. Sean's own feelings of excitement continued to build as he got into Portland and closer to Emanuel Hospital. He had his bag packed, a pillow from home, and flowers for his wife, whom he missed more than he would have ever thought.

Andrea was looking out the window with the video camera poised and ready when Sean pulled into the parking lot. She wasn't sure whether he would drive the car or the truck, and both vehicles they had were so common, she wanted to be sure it was him. He pulled up in her gold car and parked directly in front of her second story window. She knew there was no way he would look up and know where she was, but she waved anyway.

A few short moments later, there was a knock on the door. Andrea had the video camera running and just waited for him

expect a miracle *149*

to come in. Sean knocked on the door again and cracked it a little bit, and Andrea said, "Hello?" with a huge smile on her face.

Before seeing whose room it was, Sean said, "Oh, I'm sorry," and closed the door while turning to find the right room. Running to the door with the video camera, taping the ground and her own two feet, Andrea said, "No, no, no. Honey, it's me."

# BEAUTY FOR ASHES

**PSALM 30:11 NIV**
You turned my wailing into dancing; you removed
my sackcloth and clothed me with joy.

As Andrea opened the door, Sean was turned with his bag and heading down the hall away from her. She said, "Honey, you had the right room."

He turned to her confused but relieved, glad his long trip was over and he could rest with Andrea. Sean handed her a blue vase of yellow flowers. After five weeks apart, it felt strange to see each other again. Andrea took a few moments to examine Sean's face, which was certainly a sight for sore eyes. The hug they shared was long and quiet, enjoying the touch and feel of each other's warmth. She showed Sean around her room, which didn't take long. He liked the idea of the in-room fridge and VCR. The bed by the window for Sean would be tested that night for his approval (or disapproval) after comparison with his previous sleeping arrangements.

Sean was famished, but the cafeteria was closed for the night. They knew there were vending machines down the hall just outside the maternity ward and also downstairs next to the entrance to the emergency room. They took a trip together downstairs and searched the few machines for snacks. They both got egg salad sandwiches, which they found questionable coming from a vending machine. Next to that was a coffee machine that also dispensed hot cocoa. They got two cups of cocoa and took their loot back to the room to settle in for the night with some TV and conversation.

Andrea's nurse saw them coming back into the maternity ward and said, "I caught you."

It was frustrating to Andrea when they treated her like an invalid.

She said to Sean, "I'm not crippled, ya know?"

On Saturday, Sean gave Andrea all of the treasures from home that she had asked for and even some she didn't. He brought a dozen of her favorite movies, a small wedding album with their picture on the front cover, and her own bathroom stuff. Her kiwi-watermelon shampoo was just what she needed. She had gotten tired of asking the nurses in San Francisco every other day for more shampoo. He also unpacked her portable stereo/CD player and CDs from her car. Sean's parents came to visit that afternoon and were glad to see everyone back in Oregon where they belonged.

Sunday was NFL game day, and Sean made a deal with Andrea that he would stay until half time, then he needed to head back home. The weekend seemed too short to both of them, but it was nice to know it would be merely five short days before they would see each other again. Sean packed his bag and Andrea walked him down to the parking lot to say good-bye. She hopped into the passenger seat and pretended to leave with him. He drove from his parking space about halfway down the parking lot and dropped her off at the automated doors. She slowly made the trip back up to the lonely confines of her room, which at least had the sweet comforts of home.

Another great surprise that day was a visit from her mom and sisters. Since Amber lived the closest, she called to see what Andrea wanted her to bring. She brought her some Gatorade and Taco Bell bean burritos. What a difference her first week in Portland made to her spirit! Though her depression wouldn't go away for a while, the deep sorrow and loneliness that filled her each day was beginning to dissipate with each visit and each hug from someone she loved.

Each week there was another ultrasound to check Thomas's growth. This one, on Wednesday, showed he wasn't growing very well. Dr. Di Federico discussed it with her and said if he didn't grow over the next couple of weeks they would consider inducing her earlier than the thirty-five weeks previously discussed. She could see Andrea's face light up with that information and said it wouldn't be much earlier if they did it at all. She was thirty-one weeks along and biding her time with little patience, the same as in San Francisco. It may have been only her ninth day in Portland, but it was her forty-ninth day total of sitting in a hospital bed, waiting for Thomas to make his appearance.

On Thursday, more visitors. Christina and Emily drove up from Stayton and kept her company for a couple of hours before heading out again. On Friday, Trisha was leaving work at Deschutes Optical early and wanted to come by to see Andrea on her way through to Vancouver. John knew the area very well since he lived in Portland before moving to Bend, so he gave Trish great directions straight to the hospital. Andrea told her where to park and how to find her. They greeted each other with huge hugs and enjoyed making each other laugh again. If there was one thing Trisha was good for, it was laughter. She would be good medicine for anybody.

Sean arrived that afternoon at about four thirty, which was a great surprise to Andrea. They revisited the halls and cafeteria together, which had the nurses all worked up again.

When they were back in her room, Andrea said to Sean, "Don't these people realize the doctors at UCSF were promoting my increased movement? They were telling me to take more

expect a miracle *153*

walks down the maternity halls and stuff. I needed to stretch my legs. I'm as stable as they come."

"Well, they're only doing their job," Sean said. "You're supposed to be on bed rest, aren't you? I just think you shouldn't get so mad."

"What would you know about sitting in bed for a month and a half with nothing to do but watch TV and play solitaire? Oh, and getting poked constantly by needles and awakened every morning at an ungodly hour? The most excitement I get is when I get taken downstairs for an ultrasound, where I get the thrill of waiting to hear what else is wrong all by myself without my husband there to support me." She couldn't hide her anger.

Sean gave her a hug.

"I can't imagine how hard it is to be stuck here day in and day out, week in and week out. We're almost there. Just hang in there a while longer."

October 12 was Saturday, and a nurse gave the couple the tour of Emanuel's NICU. During the tour, Andrea was again irritated when the nurse made her ride in a wheelchair pushed by Sean. She had to continually stand up anyway to see what the nurse was talking about. They made their way through the labor ward, and the nurse showed them the two rooms that were closest to the resuscitation room. Since they would be delivering a high-risk premature baby, they would be directly across from where Thomas would be going immediately after birth. That would enable them to provide any necessary life support he might need.

They went through two large doors, which led to the highest-risk area of the Neonatal Intensive Care Unit. Each baby in that room had a nurse dedicated to them twenty-four hours a day. Those were extremely ill babies—the sickest of the sick. To the left, they entered a much larger area that was divided into sections. The first section was where babies had one nurse to two babies, babies which needed continual care. In the next area they were shown a baby who weighed three and a half pounds, the approximate weight of their own little guy. The biggest thing they both noticed about a baby that size was that they were just skin and bones. Tiny little people who didn't get the chance to put on all of their baby fat before coming into this world. The baby was also enveloped by many IV's and lines coming from numerous machines around the bed. Again, not a shocking sight, since they were already aware of what to expect, but it was good to get the lay of the land.

On Sunday, day fifty-three, the two of them did quite a bit more walking than Andrea had done in a very long time. After Sean hit the road, Andrea noticed all through the night that she was having a lot more contractions than before. She started to really think about what it would be like when labor actually began—something she hadn't had the chance to give much thought to. She was trying to get past one hurdle at a time. It was a good feeling to know that, when labor was confirmed, Sean was only three hours away. She no longer had lingering concerns for the life and health of her baby. He was thirty-two weeks. It was a miracle that he had made it that far. Most parents would be devastated to have their baby delivered two months early, but to Sean and Andrea, it was more than they could have ever asked for. All tests were showing only positive results for Thomas and his future. Concerns about his leg would just have to wait until after he was born, because they had already taken advantage of all that modern medicine had to offer him. All they could do was hope for the best.

During the following week, April and Andrea were on the phone together a lot. April was taking her maternity leave and being induced on Tuesday. April's doctors were concerned about the large size of her baby and were conflicted about

expect a miracle *155*

whether to deliver her early or wait. The baby wasn't due until the end of the month. It was all for naught anyway, because the pills she was given two days in a row to soften the cervix didn't take effect the way they had hoped. April was absolutely crushed when they told her to wait out the weekend and they would try again on Monday.

Andrea said, "Well, I'm pretty busy up here, but why don't you come visit me?"

April decided it would be a great way to pass the time. Again, they first discussed what food to bring, because that was the most important thing. It was Taco Bell for Andrea and Arby's for April. They sat close together and watched the video taken during the time in San Francisco on Andrea's video camera. It was very redundant, and Andrea realized that almost everyday Sean would look out the window with the camera getting the view of the bay she stared at for forty days.

She said, "If I never watch that video again, I will still never get the image of that bridge out of my head!"

April just laughed. That afternoon they watched *The Wedding Planner*, and then April went home to wait out the long weekend that would inevitably have to pass before she could say hello to her baby.

On Friday, October 18, Sean came early again, which made Andrea's day. She walked down to the cafeteria with him to get some dinner so they could eat their meals together. She wasn't being bothered by nurses anymore when she walked because she talked to one of her doctors who wrote in her chart, *Patient can walk around*. A small, but significant battle won.

Later that evening, they got egg salad sandwiches and hot cocoa from the vending machine by the emergency room. Andrea noticed her hips ached as she walked around and then all throughout the evening. Sean wanted to strangle her as she got up every hour through the night to go to the bathroom.

Before dawn Saturday morning, Andrea could barely see the clock but decided to attempt to time her contractions. They weren't painful, but seemed steady. Those were moments she had dreamed of all her life. The excitement of waking her husband up in the middle of the night, counting contractions, and debating about how soon to go the hospital. Obviously, getting to the hospital wasn't a concern in the current situation, which was just another thing Andrea was bitter about. Her experience was nothing like she had dreamed. She was already in the hospital. She didn't need to worry about how close the contractions were. The clock was nearly impossible to see in the dark room, but she thought they were about ten minutes apart.

At about six o'clock, she called a nurse in and told her she should probably be put on a monitor. After a while, the nurse came back in and checked the printed strip from the machine. Her contractions were three to four minutes apart. Yay! The nurse was followed by a resident and another nurse with a flashlight. She wanted to check Andrea's cervix visually, not by hand, to maintain a sterile environment. It wasn't wise to risk contaminating the baby by checking manually. Andrea, who was uncomfortable with the whole situation (remember, *butts are private!*) said, "Does it take three people?"

They looked at her a bit surprised and the resident said, "Well, I would like some help."

Andrea kept the serious look on her face and stood her metaphorical ground. One nurse reluctantly left the room. The resident tried to check while the nurse held the flashlight for her to see better. Andrea appeared to be three centimeters dilated. She was thrilled. By seven they had been moved to the labor and delivery side of the floor into room number one, which was directly across from the resuscitation room. Dr. Weick checked her for real that time and determined that she was four centimeters.

expect a miracle  *157*

"You are officially in labor," he said.

Sean called his parents and Andrea called April.

"I win."

April said, "What?"

"I'm in labor and you have to wait until Monday. Ha ha."

"You suck," said April, "I'll be there later, you brat."

PSALM 116:8–9 NIV

For you, O Lord, have delivered my soul from death,
my eyes from tears, my feet from stumbling, That I may
walk before the Lord in the land of the living.

Family members slowly started to trickle into the hospital. First Sean's parents, then April, followed by Amber and Steve and Mary. Being as small as Thomas was, it was supposed to be a quick, easy delivery. The doctor had told Sean and Andrea that they wouldn't even have to dilate to ten centimeters as most moms do. Everybody was there by noon and started talking about what to do about lunch. It was quite cruel since Andrea wasn't allowed to eat anything. People headed down to the cafeteria and got taco salads, brought their food back up to the room, and played cards, while Andrea sat in bed having contractions. Sean had also stopped by the gift shop and brought Andrea a stuffed lemur with a long ringed tail.

The contractions weren't very painful, but they were starting to get closer together and more intense. Once she was checked by the doctor and it was determined she was six centimeters, it was actually going really well. She thought, *Wow, maybe I could even do this without pain medication.*

But she knew that if she waited too long for pain medication, they could tell her it was too late and then she'd be up a creek without a paddle. So, even though she was still pretty

158 andrea merkord

comfortable, she decided to have the epidural placed and they called the anesthesiologist to put it in.

Having the epidural did slow down the contractions a little bit but not too much. The doctor came in a while later and increased the dose of Potosin Andrea was being given to help speed up the contractions and get things going again. The family started debating about how long it would be until the baby was delivered, making bets about what time Thomas would be born. Most of the times people were guessing were between three and four that afternoon. Four o'clock came and went, but by five o'clock, Andrea was ready to start pushing. She had already made it clear to her nurse that she wanted the least amount of people in the room as necessary. She knew there would have to be an extra nurse in there ready to take Thomas away as soon as he was born, but that was her limit.

She wasn't quite sure what to think about the experience. It wasn't like she had imagined it. She thought she would go through all these steps she had read in books and be prepared for the next step. She just wasn't really sure what to expect. She, of course, kicked everyone in the family out of the room because *butts are private*. But as they were kicking everyone out, she stopped and said, "Well, April, since I know you're about to go through this in another day or two, you can stay in here."

April took pictures while Sean's mom video taped. It had been decided previously that Carol would be the designated videographer. She taped the delivery, with a side view, of course.

Delivery was easy for Andrea, painless up until the very last moment. After only seconds of pain, suddenly Thomas was out and being laid across her belly at five thirty five PM. She was looking down at him in awe, holding her hands out to her sides, too afraid to touch him because she didn't want to inter-

expect a miracle   *159*

fere with what the doctors needed to do. She knew he was still in a very risky situation and had to be taken out of the room immediately.

However, before the doctor took him away, he did say, "Go ahead and hold his head up," while he was busy cutting the cord.

It felt strange for her to touch Thomas and cup his head in her hand. It was a moment that would be forever burned into her memory. Then he was whisked away. Thomas weighed three pounds fifteen and a half ounces, barely shy of four pounds. He was a whopping sixteen and one half inches long.

Minutes after Thomas was taken away and Andrea was alone, forgotten by everyone who was outside waiting to take turns to see Thomas, she had a single thought that subdued the excitement across the hall ... *It's over. I'm not pregnant anymore.*

She couldn't believe they arrived at that day after all. She hadn't even cried yet. Tears quickly came the moment April brought back the video camera and Andrea finally heard the wonderful sound of her own son crying and breathing on his own. Thomas felt out of reach. She couldn't hold him yet and counted the minutes until she would hold him close.

When Sean and Andrea had time alone, they spent the evening with Thomas. The nurse helped them give Thomas his first bath. They were surprised at how rough she was being with the brush on Thomas's head. He was still covered with a sticky white substance because of his prematurity, and she was trying to get it out of his hair. Andrea inspected Thomas's ankle, which still had massive scarring and constriction, but a beautiful foot with all five toes. She noticed his left wrist. There was a light band of tissue blended into his own skin, loosely wrapped around it. Sean was right when he saw the band on ultrasound! How lucky was Thomas?

160   andrea merkord

Andrea took the opportunity that night to do something every pregnant woman dreams of, sleep on her stomach. It was the most peaceful rest she had ever experienced. No nurses came in to take her blood pressure and temperature in the wee hours of the night. However, first thing in the morning, her day nurse came in bright and early and immediately started putting on gloves and reaching for Andrea's covers.

Andrea said, "What are you doing?"

The nurse said, "Checking for hemorrhoids."

Andrea quickly piped up, "I don't have any."

The nurse looked at her for a moment until she realized Andrea wasn't going to budge. She left the room unhappy with Andrea.

Sean and Andrea had to become accustomed to the routines of the Neonatal Intensive Care Unit. In the NICU, sanitation was of the utmost importance and visitors were limited. On Sunday, the doctor told her that she could be discharged the following day or she could stay a day longer if they wanted to be close to Thomas.

Andrea quickly responded, "You can discharge me tomorrow."

Sixty-one days. That would be the final tally. Sixty-one days in a hospital bed. Who could have guessed? That number would forever be branded into Andrea's memory. Sixty-one days.

Preparing to leave Thomas was torturous. They wondered what they were thinking when they planned to go home without him. Transport arrangements would be made for Thomas as soon as he was able and as soon as medical transport could be arranged from Portland to Bend (déjà vu). It was Monday, October 21. As Andrea was packing her bags to leave that day, it was strange to feel so excited to be leaving, but so sad at the same time, to be leaving Thomas behind. They hurriedly

expect a miracle *161*

packed the bags onto a cart they could wheel out to the car. As they were heading to the elevator, Dr. Merrill, one of the perinatologists, stopped her and kind of joked, "I'm sorry, but I think we're gonna have to keep you a little longer."

Andrea turned around, pretending to run away, and said, "I don't think so. I have plotted my escape."

Once the car was packed and they were ready to go, they went back upstairs to give Thomas another feeding and find some way inside themselves to say good-bye and trust that he would be well taken care of while they were away. Andrea planned to come back in a day or two, but it was still so much harder to say good-bye than she thought it would be. She needed to head home, and she knew she couldn't afford to stay in Portland any longer. In the car on the way down the interstate, they heard a song by Michelle Branch, "Good-bye to You," that made Andrea cry and cry.

They knew that morning that April had been admitted to the Stayton hospital so she could finally deliver her own precious baby. Sean and Andrea made a point to go home on Highway 22 via Stayton so they could stop by the hospital and possibly see the baby, or at least say hello. When they got there, April was just getting started and getting hooked up with her epidural. Since it would still be a long evening before a new baby arrived, Andrea and Sean hit the road for the two-hour drive home. It was a good thing they didn't wait it out. It wasn't until after ten o'clock that Morgan Paige joined the family at eight pounds twelve ounces, two days after her cousin.

When they got back into Bend, Andrea could not believe how much it had changed in a two-month period. They joked that it was the construction capital of the world, but she realized how true that was when the city seemed to have changed through the summer. One of the large billboards as they entered town had changed to a completely different advertisement, so that threw her for a loop. When they got farther into town and around the corner from their townhouse, there was a gigantic retirement home that had been built. She said, "Holy cow, where'd that monstrosity come from?"

Sean looked at her and, as innocently as could be, said, "Where have you been?"

They both just stopped and laughed at that comment. Coming home was surreal. No one thinks they're going to come home without their baby. It felt like something was missing. It was nice to see her cat, Hanna, who seemed confused at seeing Andrea again. They talked to the nurses in the NICU that night and the doctor and found that Thomas was doing just fine. They could call whenever they wanted while they were away to hear how he was doing.

### 1 JOHN 4:4 NIV

You, dear children, are from God and have overcome them, because the one who is in you is greater than the one who is in the world.

Andrea settled in back at home easily. Monday morning, she called John, who congratulated her on her new arrival. John made a strange statement to her that she wasn't quite sure how to take.

He said, "Well, I'm not sure what to do with you."

She was ready to go back to work, so she waited and let the day go by, expecting him to call back and tell her to come into work, but the call didn't come.

On Tuesday, she finally called him a little bit upset and said, "I came home so I could go to work, otherwise I would have just stayed up in Portland."

He said, "Oh, I didn't realize that. Let me figure out what the plan is here now and I'll call you back."

She was very frustrated and actually getting a little wor-

expect a miracle   *163*

ried that John wasn't going to bring her back or was replacing her. She didn't know what to think. So she decided Tuesday afternoon that when Sean got up for work on Wednesday, she would get up bright and early and spend the day with Thomas. She made it there around eleven for his feeding and got to spend several hours with him. It was so wonderful to sit there with him quietly by herself.

The hospital gave breastfeeding moms a voucher for lunch in the cafeteria, which made it nice for her, so she didn't have to buy lunch. Leaving again that afternoon was difficult, but she knew she would be back on the weekend to see him, which comforted her. She was glad she was able to come during the week and spend some time with him. She was still hoping to go back to work so she could pass the time and not wait at home for the day Thomas would come home.

On Thursday morning, the phone rang around nine o'clock and it was Trisha.

She said, "What are you doing?"

Andrea said, "Well, I'm getting Thomas's room ready for him since I didn't have time to do that before."

Trisha said, "Get in here!"

Andrea was happy to have something to do to pass the time and hopped in the shower, got dressed, and headed into work. People didn't ask too much about what had gone on with her or what she had been doing. She was pretty sure they had been told not to ask her about it.

Friday, October 25, Sean and Andrea drove to Albany after work to stay at Sean's parents' house for the weekend so they could drive up to see Thomas in Portland. Andrea wanted so badly to go to the hospital Friday night, but Sean didn't feel like driving up for one feeding, driving back down, and turning around and driving back up again in the morning. He wanted to just go up for the eleven o'clock feeding Saturday morning.

Andrea decided that since she was so eager to see Thomas, she would get up very early to be at the hospital for his eight AM feeding. That way she could spend some time with him alone before large numbers of family members came to visit him. She got the chance to practice his routine by checking his temperature under his armpit, changing his tiny preemie diaper, and getting him all bundled up and ready for his feeding.

After his feeding, she held him for at least an hour and a half, just rocking him in the rocking chair. She got him all wrapped up again and put him back into his isolette so she could go outside and get ready for Sean and his parents to arrive. They had other visitors that day too. Karla came. Craig and Tandi came. Sean's cousin, James, who was living in Portland at the time, stopped by to take some pictures and e-mail them back to his parents, who lived in Georgia. With all the commotion that morning, Thomas was having trouble dealing with the excess stimulation and his heart rate kept dropping to dangerous levels. Andrea had a hard time dealing with that.

Everyone decided to go out to a Mexican restaurant for lunch. Andrea couldn't get Thomas out of her mind. She felt so guilty about the visitation. It had been too much for him to handle, and she had to excuse herself from the table to go to the bathroom, where she cried some more. She felt guilty for stimulating him too much by holding him that morning. It wasn't fair that she couldn't even hold her son without problems arising. Sean and Andrea spent more time at the hospital that afternoon with Thomas and returned to Albany that evening to sleep, but they got up bright and early Sunday morning, went back up to the hospital, spent the day with Thomas, and drove home Sunday afternoon.

The following week actually passed fairly quickly, considering they didn't go to visit Thomas Monday through Friday, which ate them both up. The fact that Andrea was going to

expect a miracle  *165*

work during the week definitely helped pass the time. They continued calling the NICU nurses and checking on Thomas to see how he was doing. Of course, the doctors who visited Thomas each day would call Andrea and give her the official update on his condition and how well he was growing. Over all, he was doing great. All he needed to do was maintain his temperature on his own, which he was very close to doing. He needed to be able to suck and swallow and have a full bottle on his own without having difficulties. He was very close to both. There was no specific weight he had to reach before he could go home. He just needed to grow up enough to maintain his heart rate, body temperature, and feed well.

### JOB 10:12 NIV
You gave me life and showed me kindness, and in
your providence watched over my spirit.

Saturday, November 1, Sean and Andrea decided to wake up early instead of driving Friday night. The three-hour drive seemed to last an eternity. The plan was to be there before eleven o'clock to feed Thomas at his regularly scheduled time. They were also meeting Andrea's parents there. When they arrived with anticipation building up inside after an exhaustive week away from Thomas, Steve and Mary were already waiting for them.

Andrea's feelings returned to childhood when she was afraid of upsetting her father. For some reason she was more concerned about making her dad wait than anything else. Because of the people limit allowed in the NICU, Andrea asked Sean if she could take her parents in first to see Thomas. She didn't realize until much later how much that upset him. He hadn't seen his own son in a week and her thoughtlessness made him wait outside longer than he should have. Her guilty feelings later made her wonder why she suddenly felt fear of upsetting her dad, who was not the same person he was when she was growing up. Was she not adult enough to understand and separate her childish feelings from the importance of her husband's needs and place him first?

While Sean and Andrea were sitting quietly with Thomas, some wonderful, but untimely news came. They had only been there for fifteen minutes when the nurse told them transport was coming to get Thomas to take him to Bend. Although the transport was what they'd been waiting for, it meant someone had to turn around and drive the car three hours right back to Bend. Sean assumed that task, and Andrea waited in Portland to ride with Thomas.

Sean was the first to arrive at St. Charles Medical Center in Bend, because arrangements in Portland for Thomas's flight were slow and drawn out, but eventually the family was together. That evening at home, Andrea felt another huge mile marker had been reached. She was less than one mile from Thomas and could go feed and hold him any time she wanted. He spent the next ten days being visited constantly by his parents and growing up so he could prepare to come home.

Sunday, November 10, at St. Charles, Thomas was moved to a room on the maternity floor to spend the night with Andrea before being discharged to go home for good. During the day, Thomas had been put through a "car seat test" to see how he did with his breathing in a semi-seated position. The doctor told Andrea that Thomas had failed the test but was being discharged anyway. Andrea wondered what the purpose of the test was if they were going to ignore the results. They had trusted medical professionals up to that point and assumed it was safe to take Thomas home if the doctor said so.

Taking Thomas home was anything but the typical new baby experience. As with all of their dealings with Thomas

expect a miracle  *167*

thus far, it was wrought with added complications. He would remain on oxygen and an apnea monitor at home and would have portable units to use when they left the house.

A very large, noisy unit was placed in Thomas's room for his permanent oxygen supply, and his apnea monitor was mostly portable until they would plug it in to recharge through the night. The lights on it would blink with his breathing and heartbeat. When his heart rate dropped too low, the alarm would sound, or if Thomas stopped breathing, the alarm would sound. It was a deafening and frightening noise for Thomas and his parents. Sean and Andrea learned how quickly they could go from dead weight on their pillows to standing at the crib side, which was directly across the hall from them.

On many occasions, Thomas would stop breathing, and Sean and Andrea would watch him turn blue as he was choking on his own vomit. They struggled to suction his nose and throat and help him to catch his breath. They would be desperately saying under their breath, "Come on. Come on. Breathe. Breathe."

When he would finally breathe and cry, it was another catastrophe averted, and Andrea would sit in the rocking chair with Thomas, tears streaming down her cheeks, while Thomas's tiny body lay limp on her shoulder, exhausted from the terrifying and confusing experiences.

Finally, the home health nurse figured out Thomas had "reflux," which was causing his vomiting, and thus the choking episodes. He was prescribed medication and rice cereal was added to his bottles, which reduced the episodes to practically nil. Sean couldn't help but wonder if Thomas should have been kept at the hospital longer. They didn't feel equipped to handle the near tragic episodes that were taking place. Sean held Andrea at night and felt angry again at how difficult and scary their parenting experience was. When would life quiet down, and when could they relax for even a moment of time? Not for quite a while, unfortunately.

Andrea did not officially begin her maternity leave until Thomas came home from the hospital. Then she stayed home for six weeks with him. Even during that leave, she felt so guilty about what a burden she had been to John that she offered to work two hours each evening to help with inventory. When Sean got home around five each afternoon, Andrea would go to work until about seven. It worked out well for Sean, who had the chance to spend time alone with his son. After the Christmas holiday, Andrea would go back full time after being gone for the past four months.

Thomas remained on oxygen until almost Christmas time and the apnea monitor until well into the New Year. On December 19, 2002, Thomas reached another big step along his dangerous path. The week before his first Christmas, he had plastic surgery on his ankle to remove the remaining scar tissue that was continuing to constrict blood flow. He had reached a whopping nine pounds by that day, two months of age, and the doctors felt he could handle the surgery. He had also reached a crucial point for his foot, which needed more blood flow.

Preparing for leg surgery was frightening for Andrea. She had this big fear of anesthesia complications with Thomas. She didn't know how he would react and until he had surgery, there would be no way to know how his body would do under anesthesia. They got to the hospital early, around six o'clock that morning, to get checked in. They got in the pre-op area, where they were given a tiny, adorable white gown with pink elephants on it. It tied behind Thomas's neck, and she looked at his little legs curled up in the fetal position. She thought he looked adorable. In that little gown he was just so cute.

She was very afraid someone was going to try to put an IV in and it would be a horrible nightmare, but luckily they didn't

expect a miracle *169*

do that. The anesthesiologist and a nurse came to get him and took him away. Luckily, he didn't cry, which helped Andrea to maintain control herself. The couple headed to the cafeteria as a way to pass some time. They had some breakfast and made their way down with their bag and Thomas's belongings to the waiting room. They left their bags at a couch and went down the hall to the gift shop and looked around to pass some more time. Andrea found a darling little orange stuffed cat she bought for Thomas for after the surgery. While they were sitting in the waiting room, Andrea was trying to talk herself up and subdue any fears she had about the surgery.

She looked at Sean and said, "Ya know, this is just a superficial surgery. It's just his skin, the outside of his body. He's gonna do just fine. It's not like it's open-heart surgery, right?"

She had this very prophetic way of putting her foot in her mouth which, of course, she did not realize at the time.

Both doctors came out to talk to them a while later to tell them that Thomas did great during the surgery. He was doing fine in the post-op area. They couldn't see him immediately though. They needed to wait until a nurse came to get them once he was revived from anesthesia. About forty-five minutes later, someone finally did come. Andrea got into the room and held him. He had this tiny, pathetic cry that was being quieted by pain meds and leftover anesthesia. It was just as Amber had described to her. Amber had warned her what it was like to have a child in surgery and told her the worst part was how pathetic they are under medication and how you want to take their pain away. In agreement with Amber, she found that to be the most difficult part of the experience.

Tears began coming from her eyes as she was holding Thomas.

The nurse looked at her and said, "It's really hard, isn't it?"

Andrea nodded her head quietly. She held Thomas as they

were wheeled to the pediatric ward, where they would spend the night. She slept in a bed next to his crib, and late during the night before she fell asleep, she heard next door a young child, maybe three or four years old. That child was having something done. She could hear maybe a mom and a nurse in there talking to her and trying to quiet her fears, but the child was crying and yelling, "No, no, no!"

Andrea imagined maybe they were trying to take blood or something. She really didn't know, but she thought about how lucky she was. How lucky she was that with as many things as Thomas had been through and as many risks that had been put to his life and his well being, he would not have any lifelong or chronic diseases or conditions or anything that would cause him to have continual pain or procedures. She just didn't think she could handle a child who had chronic illness. It would break her heart. It would absolutely break her heart.

She was reminded again how, although their experiences were so difficult, they were actually very lucky to have gone through them, because they had the opportunity, unlike a lot of parents, to treasure their child for who he was and how lucky he was to be there and not take him for granted. He hadn't come easy. He had a rough beginning, and they were lucky to realize how wonderful it was to have him in their lives.

On a wonderful Saturday afternoon, Dr. Farmer from UCSF, who was visiting Central Oregon, came by to see Thomas. It was so generous of her to spend her own time to visit with them. She had a picture taken while she held Thomas to take back with her to UCSF. Unfortunately, she couldn't see how his leg turned out, because he was still in a cast from plastic surgery. Andrea was able to find a picture of Thomas to give her though. In it, you could see his mangled ankle pretty well.

With 2003 coming in, Sean and Andrea looked forward to the New Year and a better future for their small family, but

expect a miracle

the time to exhale had not yet come. After persevering through their unbelievable troubles, there was one more hurdle to cross. One more unexpected turn of events that was cruel and unfair to precious little Thomas and his weary parents.

MATTHEW 11:28 NIV

Come to me, all who are weary and burdened, and I will give you rest.

# A PROMISE KEPT

**2 CORINTHIANS 4:17–18 NIV**

*For our light and momentary troubles are achieving for us an eternal glory that far outweighs them all. So we fix our eyes not on what is seen, but on what is unseen. For what is seen is temporary, but what is unseen is eternal.*

They entered the New Year with hopes of putting 2002 behind them and becoming a healthy, happy family once and for all. Andrea's maternity leave officially ended on Christmas Eve, so she had a daycare provider ready to go to start watching Thomas. She went against her gut instinct and took him to a home with which she wasn't one hundred percent comfortable. She told herself she was being paranoid and Thomas would be fine. After four long days, and a mishap with Thomas's monitor, Andrea took Thomas out of her care without any idea of who would watch him while she worked.

The most timely opportunity came when Sean asked his dad to spend the week at their house watching Thomas during the day. Tony was more than happy to oblige. After one week of that, Andrea used the same idea and asked her sister to pitch in. April took turns with Tony and spent the next week of her maternity leave not only taking care of her newborn, but Andrea's as well. That trade went on for about a month.

Finally, neither of them could keep spending weeks in Bend with Thomas; Sean and Andrea had to make a decision. Andrea didn't have the heart to drop Thomas off at another daycare yet and went into John's office with a proposal. John was quick to give Andrea permission to set up her work space with a playpen and bouncy seat for Thomas. More than anything John ever did for her, that was the most generous and selfless thing he could have done at the time. It was fun for her to sit at her desk working and look up to her right, where Thomas slept in his bouncy seat peacefully next to her. She had the best of both worlds. After a while, Sean finally found a home daycare mom who had three children of her own and would only be adding Thomas to the mix. It was what they wanted, and Amy was the perfect provider for Thomas's needs.

When Thomas got sick, they didn't want to overreact with any possible sign of illness, but then again, with a preemie, you can't be too careful. When he started coughing, they figured they'd keep an eye on him and see what happened; but after about a week, they decided to take him in and get it checked out. They took him to the doctor after work around seven o'clock on a snowy January night. It turned out they were lucky; Dr. Chunn was the person on call that night. They hadn't met him yet, but they had to be seen by who was on call. He listened to Thomas's chest and didn't seem too concerned about the cough as long as it hadn't been accompanied by anything else.

As he listened he said, "Well, I don't know this little guy very well, but he has a heart murmur, right?"

Andrea looked at him with a wrinkled brow.

"No."

"Well, he does," the doctor said very matter-of-factly as he continued to listen. "Yeah, it's definitely there."

He told them they needed to schedule a cardiac echo in the next day or two. If they contacted his nurse in the morning, she would get it set up. That night they called a couple of family members and gave them the latest news. They all knew a lot of babies born with heart murmurs would grow out of them with no problems as a result of ever having one. It was still a frightening concept. All they could do was wait until morning.

When Andrea got to work, she told the people in the office she would be scheduling another appointment because Thomas had a heart murmur.

They all said the same thing she already knew, "Most murmurs are nothing to worry about."

Andrea just shook her head and said, "Look at the last seven months. Have we gotten off that easy with anything? No. Of course not. With Thomas it's been, *what can go wrong will go wrong!*" She started to cry.

Memories came rushing back to Andrea as she sat in the visitors chair at work. Remembering the day after an ultrasound when she came back and told coworkers that the membranes were no longer in tact and the doctor couldn't tell them what it meant. It could have been nothing or everything. Of course, it became everything. That parallel situation was as volatile. The heart murmur could be nothing or everything. Sean and Andrea had been trained to expect the worst possible news and both had a bad feeling about the latest situation.

After Thomas had his echo on that sunny, but cold January afternoon, Sean and Andrea waited with him in a patient room to talk to the pediatric cardiologist about the results. Dr. Tajchman was a young female doctor, and Andrea thought she couldn't have been much older than her own twenty-eight years. She was very gentle in the way she spoke. She told them Thomas did have a condition called Pulmonary Stenosis, where the pulmonary artery had a narrowing point in the artery and in the valve itself, which would eventually require surgery. During the echo, they had been measuring the amount of pressure it was taking to get the blood through the artery and valve. Anything over twenty was a mild case, anything over

expect a miracle *175*

forty was a moderate case, and over sixty was severe. Thomas measured about sixty-five.

Dr. Tajchman told them the condition was a progressive one—that would start out mild and increase to a higher level until it became too constrictive and would require surgical repair. Andrea wondered to herself how it could possibly already be severe when no other doctor had ever mentioned that he had anything close to a heart murmur. Thank goodness for Dr. Chunn. Dr. Tajchman gave them pamphlets about what it would be like to have open-heart surgery and what they could expect with recovery time. The pamphlet included information on what it involves when doctors put patients on the heart-lung machine during the procedure and how the surgery is performed. The doctor told them to come back in two weeks. Andrea read and re-read every pamphlet she was given.

Andrea took Thomas to the next appointment herself and tried to watch the screen. It was totally opposite of her knowing what to look at on the ultrasound screens. She couldn't tell what they were looking at, what they were looking for, or what they were measuring. She sat there just waiting to find out if the pressure had increased. When the doctor came in to talk to her, the pressure had increased somewhat, but not as much as she had expected. Dr. Tajchman told her that she had expected a much larger increase in pressure between appointments, considering how suddenly the condition had appeared in the first place. She told them the number would need to be over eighty or eighty-five for it to require surgery, and she set them up for a return appointment in a month. It was best to allow Thomas to get as big and strong as possible before his surgery, which is why they would postpone it as long as possible.

Waiting out another month was draining. Sean couldn't have been happier. He wanted to let it go as long as possible and put it off as long as they could. He did not want to face that surgery. Andrea, on the other hand, had a completely opposite perspective. She couldn't stand the waiting, and it was eating at her every day. She would have rather gotten it over with just so they could get it behind them and finally move on.

During the time of just waiting before surgery, Sean's dad would call every night and see how Thomas was doing. Everyone in the family always knew when Thomas had an appointment, so they either waited for their phone call or called to find out what the results of any given test were. Sean's dad, on the other hand, called everyday, all the time, and it was driving Andrea crazy. They had spent the previous year giving every detail of their lives to everybody they knew, and she was so tired of it. She just wanted a time of peace and quiet to live a life with their new little family without reporting every detail anymore.

On the other side of the spectrum, Andrea wished her parents had called more often. Of course, Andrea's expectations were never really clear to anybody. Sean and Andrea wanted to pick and choose when they wanted people to be there for them and when they wanted them to leave them alone, so truth be told, that wasn't fair to anybody else either. It would have been nice to have a happy medium from both sides.

One night, Sean's sister, Karla, called, and Andrea happened to be the one who answered the phone. She was very frustrated and tired of all the struggles they had gone through.

Karla sensed that as she was talking to Andrea and said, "People are praying for Thomas and praying he gets better."

Andrea very quickly blurted out, "He's not getting better. It is a progressive condition that will get worse until it requires surgery."

Karla was shocked at how quickly Andrea had come back with that, but Andrea was so frustrated at people not under-

expect a miracle  *177*

standing what the situation was when she had explained it very clearly.

Andrea handed the phone to Sean, and Karla said to him, "Boy, it sure doesn't sound like Andrea's having very much faith."

Sean explained that Andrea was very tired of the ongoing problems, and she was also stressed about the upcoming surgery.

After Sean hung up the phone with Karla, he told Andrea what she had said about her not appearing to have much faith.

Andrea became upset at that comment and looked at Sean and said, "You know, I didn't get here to where we are today without faith! My faith is strong enough to move mountains, and I believe God could literally move a mountain if he wanted to. I believe God could save Thomas if he wants to, but I also believe he doesn't have to. It's not a lack of faith in God. Faith is not the absence of fear. It's the knowledge I have that God doesn't have to save Thomas's life."

Sean totally understood where Andrea was coming from and told her not to get upset at Karla for making a comment she didn't mean anything by. There had been numerous occasions when people were trying to help but just didn't understand where they were coming from.

### HEBREWS 11:1 NIV
Now faith is being sure of what we hope for
and certain of what we do not see.

At the next month's echo, Andrea had learned when to see the numbers on the screen that reflected the pressure they were measuring, and that time it read one hundred and five, which was well above the number the doctor had given them that would require surgery. The doctor came in very shortly after that and sat down on the edge of the ultrasound table and said, "Well, you probably saw where the number was."

Andrea nodded her head.

The doctor continued, "It's time to go ahead and schedule his surgery."

She said she would contact the surgeons in Portland and they would start getting it arranged for sometime in the next couple of weeks. Andrea told Sean that afternoon that surgery was imminent. He wasn't surprised but was disappointed they had to face surgery so soon.

Andrea received a call a day later from people in Portland who would assist in scheduling the surgery. The surgery was set for Friday, March 28, 2003. That was two weeks away, and it became very real to her all of a sudden what they were going to have to go through. Sean, as usual, was the travel agent of the family and arranged some hotels where they could stay in Portland so that they could be close to Thomas the entire time.

When Andrea went back to work, she told them the specific days she would need off for Thomas's surgery but didn't know how long she would be off after the surgery, possibly just a few days. Trisha walked up to where Andrea was standing and hopped up onto a table next to Andrea's computer. She was very curious about the whole process. She had a scared look on her face and asked, "Andrea, what's gonna happen to him? What are they gonna do?"

Andrea proceeded to tell what the pamphlet said the procedure was like, what they used to open up the rib cage, how they hooked him up to the heart-lung machine, and what recovery would be like. Trisha couldn't even fathom what it would be like to watch her own son go through that type of surgery and asked Andrea, "How are you gonna handle that?"

expect a miracle *179*

Andrea just shook her head and said, "I don't know. If I could take his place, I would."

Trisha said, "I know you would."

Andrea made an appointment to get photos of Thomas taken that week. There was an unspoken urgency, understood between she and Sean, that it was important to have those pictures taken. Of course, they were purchasing a package deal, and when they were offered the chance to purchase extra poses, they didn't pass that up.

Wednesday night, March 26, they drove to Albany to spend the night. It was a familiar feeling to be there in anticipation of an upcoming medical procedure. On Thursday morning, they checked into the hospital in the same diagnostic area they knew well. They had to go to an area down the hall where a lady took all of Thomas's information and weighed him. They noticed her hand was a little bit misshapen, and she saw in Thomas's chart that he had amniotic band syndrome at his left ankle.

The nurse said, "He had amniotic band syndrome."

Andrea said, "He sure did."

The nurse said, "That's what happened to my hand when I was a baby."

They found a little common ground there.

They were told to report upstairs with lab orders to have Thomas's blood drawn for a large amount of pre-op blood work that needed to be done before the next day. It was something Andrea had been dreading. She hated needles and didn't want Thomas to go through having his blood drawn. She had no idea how awful it would actually be though.

They lay Thomas on this small table and the nurse needed to wrap him up in a pillowcase. It did a good job of holding his arms to his sides so she could have access to his forearms and the inside of his elbows to access veins. Thomas hated the constriction and started crying immediately. As soon as the nurse started poking him with the needle, he started screaming at the top of his lungs, and Andrea had the unfortunate duty of being the one who was holding him still. She wanted so badly to just cuddle him, but she was using all of her energy to hold him down because he was so strong.

Sean absolutely hated the whole experience and left the room. The nurse couldn't get that vein and tried again and didn't get the next one. Another nurse came into the room, and eventually there were three nurses in there who had all tried veins in Thomas's arms.

Andrea picked him up and said, "Stop! How many times are you gonna keep trying? That is enough."

They all looked at each other and the first nurse said, "Well, I tried two times."

The next nurse said, "I tried at least two times."

The third nurse said, "Well, I tried two times."

Andrea said, "Well, that is too much."

The third nurse, who looked like she was a little more experienced, said, "Okay. Let me try *one* more time."

As difficult as it was for Andrea, she continued to hold him down because she wanted to be close to him. The other nurses were standing close, helping to hold his legs still. She attempted to find a vein on the left side of Thomas's head above his ear. She found a vein and got a good amount of blood from it. Enough that they could do the majority of the pre-op blood work. Andrea was crying by the time it was done and she wrapped Thomas in his blanket. He fell asleep on her shoulder, completely worn out from straining and crying. It was the single most heartbreaking experience she had had up to that point.

After that *delightful* experience, they were sent upstairs to the cardiologist's office, which, strangely enough, was very

expect a miracle

close to the perinatologist's office. They saw Dr. McIrvin, who explained to them what the procedure would be like. They would take a small piece of Thomas's own tissue from the pericardium and they would cut open the artery and valve and patch it with that material to create a wider opening. They also had a meeting with the surgeon, Dr. Starr, at the same time, and he discussed the procedure again. He was pleasant to talk to, very professional. They had some of their fears calmed.

Dr. McIrvin asked if they had any other questions, and Andrea said, "So, if *something* does happen to Thomas, will I get to hold him afterward?"

He looked at her with this look on his face like he was either trying to get her to spit it out or clarify what she was asking.

She said frankly, "If he dies, can I hold him?"

He nodded his head and said, "Yes, of course you could."

### 2 CORINTHIANS 1:9–10 NIV

Indeed, in our hearts we felt the sentence of death. But this happened that we might not rely on ourselves but on God, who raises the dead. He has delivered us from such a deadly peril, and he will deliver us. On him we have set our hope that he will continue to deliver us.

They went to their hotel and settled in for the night, trying to prepare themselves for the next morning. They were given some special soap and were told to give Thomas a very thorough bath. They did that and took some pictures of him out of his bath and just spent time with him. Amber stopped by the hotel room to visit with him a little bit. She gave Andrea some money for her birthday, which was that upcoming Saturday. Amber told her she wanted them to buy themselves a scanner/printer so they could e-mail pictures of Thomas to her as he grew.

They woke up very early so they could pack up their bags; they would be staying at a different hotel for the remainder of the time in Portland. They weren't allowed to give Thomas a feeding that morning, which Andrea was very concerned about. She thought if he was crying from hunger, it would make it harder for her to hand him over to the nurse when that frightful time came. He was wonderful throughout the morning. It was a gift from God that he was peaceful and quiet. He was wrapped in his blanket, and she held him while he slept the whole morning, which was very unlike him. He was an early morning, early feeding baby, and she was so surprised and so thankful for that gift.

In the pre-op area, the nurse offered a pastor to them for support and they agreed. He came up and said a prayer with them. Sean and Andrea both had tears running down their cheeks throughout the prayer, and they were starting to get nervous about handing their son over to a stranger. As Andrea started lifting her arms to hand Thomas over to the nurse, she started taking his blanket off to take his personal stuff with her, and the nurse said, "You can send that in there with him if you want to."

Andrea loved the idea that he could have his own blanket, and she left him wrapped up in it and handed him over to the nurse. Thomas didn't open his eyes or make a sound. Andrea was just in awe of how wonderful he was.

They watched the nurse carry him through a set of double doors, and they walked out another set of double doors. They just kind of stood there for a moment, looking at each other, not wanting to cry. They both stifled their tears and did what they normally did, which was head to the cafeteria to start passing the time with food. Sean and Andrea had specifically

expect a miracle *183*

asked family members not to show up early that morning so they could have time with Thomas themselves. They wanted to have that morning with Thomas before he went into surgery without anybody else around.

April was the first to arrive at around nine o'clock. She found them upstairs at the patient waiting area just outside of the pediatric ICU area. While they were visiting, their main nurse contact for the day came up to tell them what was going on during the surgery. She was the person who was designated to go into the O.R. periodically, get an update on his situation, and then go back upstairs to the patient waiting area and let the family know how the patient was doing during the long surgery. As soon as she came in the room, all talking stopped and all eyes were on her until she was done stating what she had to say.

She told Sean and Andrea Thomas was doing fine, he was on the heart-lung machine, and things were going the way they were supposed to be going. It would be several hours before he was out though.

April ran down to her car to get *Trivial Pursuit*, the game she had brought to play with Andrea while they waited. Sean was sitting quietly on the couch while the girls played their intense trivia game. Soon, Sean's parents arrived to hang out until Thomas came out of surgery. The nurse came in around ten o'clock to give them another update. Thomas was doing well, and everyone was able to exhale again and keep hoping he would continue to do great throughout the rest of the procedure.

The pastor from a church they had been attending in Bend happened to be in Portland for the weekend. He stopped by the hospital to say hello to them. The family stood in a circle, held hands, and said a prayer for Thomas that he would have a speedy recovery. At ten forty, the nurse surprised Sean and

*184* andrea merkord

Andrea by coming into the room to give them an update. They weren't expecting her until eleven o'clock, and Sean's heart stopped. He was so, so afraid she was coming in with bad news. She actually came in to tell them Thomas was already being disconnected from the heart-lung machine. He was doing awesome and would be heading upstairs in a little over an hour. The nurse told them they could stand outside of the ICU area in the hall and they could watch as Thomas was taken by on his bed into the ICU. They wouldn't be allowed in the ICU yet, but they would get the chance to see him on the way by.

When the nurse left the waiting room after giving the update, Sean completely broke down and started crying.

Andrea moved closer to him and rubbed his back, asking, "Were you afraid she was coming in with bad news?"

All Sean could get out of his mouth was, "Yeah."

April stood by just imagining how hard it was for those two parents to go through another horrifying procedure.

So they went out into the hall and waited for Thomas to come by. They knew it would be a good fifteen minutes before he would come, but April was ready with the video camera. Andrea wanted April to get a view of him going by.

Sean and Andrea waited and waited, then someone ahead of the bed came down the hall and said, "He's on his way."

Andrea jumped up and ran to the area of the hallway in front of the entrance to the ICU. They could see his bed coming. The nurse was handling things around Thomas. With tons of wires and tubes, they almost couldn't see a little baby in there. There was an anesthesiologist who was pumping an air bag into Thomas's nose and mouth, breathing for him on his trip to the ICU, so there was no time to stop and talk. The doctors needed to get him hooked up to the equipment in the ICU. They told Sean and Andrea, on their way by, that Thomas was doing wonderfully and they would be able to see him shortly.

expect a miracle  *185*

Dr. Starr came by on his way through and explained to Sean and Andrea that he actually thought something with the surgery was kind of weird. It seemed as though there was something wrapped around the artery. Some tissue or something. He said it was very rare.

Sean and Andrea just looked at each other, both of them thinking, *Of course it was rare. We would expect no less.*

Later, they would ask Dr. McIrvin about that. They asked what he thought about the idea of something being wrapped around the artery, and he looked at them with a very confused look on his face like, *What are you talking about?*

They both very specifically remembered Dr. Starr saying that. It was kind of weird.

They went back to the waiting area because they knew they wouldn't be allowed in to see Thomas for a while. Karla came with a bag of birthday gifts for Andrea. While Andrea was looking through them and looking at a bear Karla brought for Thomas, the nurse came into the room and said, "Would you like to go see him?"

Andrea dropped what she had in her hand so she and Sean could go immediately. Seeing Thomas hooked up to what appeared to be an endless number of tubes and machines, drains and catheters, unconscious, with a breathing tube in his mouth, wasn't as shocking as one might think. It was still difficult to see the red, bloody wound on his chest that was open to the air. They talked to him, touched his head, and held his hand. It was nice because he had his own blanket covering his legs to give him a feeling of comfort. He was under heavy sedation, though, so he was asleep the majority of the time.

All afternoon Friday, various visitors came in and out. Some people did okay with it and took pictures with Thomas and talked to him. Other family members had a very hard time seeing him that way and quickly left the room. Andrea brought headphones, CDs, drinks, and books, with plans to spend a lot of time waiting in that room next to Thomas, passing the hours.

Sean and Andrea went to another hotel Friday night and checked in after giving the ICU nurse all of their information, which she wrote on a magic erase board on the wall with all of his pertinent information. Getting rest came easily because they were exhausted from the previous two days, and they knew they were right around the corner from the hospital if anyone needed them. They went back to the hospital early Saturday and did the same routine. Spent time with Thomas, headed to the cafeteria, and visited with family members. Andrea's parents came to see Thomas that day and spent a good amount of time in the hall chit-chatting. Just as in the Neonatal ICU, the pediatric ICU also had a limit of two people in the room at a time, so visits had to be coordinated well.

Saturday, being Andrea's twenty-ninth birthday, she was sad that she hadn't had the chance to actually hold Thomas since before the surgery. Tony and Carol had come that afternoon. Amber also stopped by as a show of support, and they all decided to go out to a nice birthday dinner. They went to a very nice restaurant in a mall not too far from the hospital. It was a pleasant, but brief escape from the helpless reality that was lying in a hospital bed not far from where they were sitting.

On Sunday morning, Andrea finally got to hold Thomas. He was being disconnected from almost all of the wires he was connected to and also the breathing tube. The doctors wanted the parents to leave the room for the removal of the breathing tube, but Andrea said, "Why? I'd rather stay."

The doctor said, "It's not very pleasant."

He said she could stand outside the door. However, when Andrea stood outside the door, the nurse shut the curtains almost all the way, and the small space Andrea could see through was being blocked by the nurse on purpose.

expect a miracle  *187*

Andrea thought to herself, *Believe me, my imagination is much worse than any reality. How bad could it possibly be?*

But in a split second's time, the tube was out and they were allowed in the room again. The nurses were actually getting Thomas ready to be transferred out of the ICU and to the pediatric ward for the next couple of days. Andrea got to give him a feeding of his bottle and cuddle him in his blanket, rocking him. She enjoyed those moments.

Andrea had seen in the Neonatal ICU that a lot of the children had personal things in their beds, and it made it more homey for them. She had planned ahead and brought stuff from Thomas's crib at home to make his crib at the hospital feel more like his own. Andrea put his own crib bumper in with the designs he was used to staring at and even a little musical fish tank that hung on the side of the crib. She would push the buttons for him so he could listen to the music that comforted him at home.

Tony and Carol came to visit again. April also came up with Morgan. April asked Andrea if she wanted to escape for a little while and go to the shopping center that was close by. Andrea asked Sean if he wouldn't mind her leaving for a while, and he said it was fine. He would stay and visit with his parents. The sisters wandered the gigantic shopping mall for a couple of hours, stopping for lunch. While they were at the Gap buying some t-shirts, April was digging through her purse and looking down at Morgan, who was smiling at her. April started talking to Morgan, making her smile and laugh. All of a sudden, Andrea felt this deep desire to be with Thomas, even though he hadn't even looked her in the eye for three days. Seeing Morgan smile at her mom made Andrea want to return to Thomas so badly that she suddenly said to April, "Let's go back after this."

Sunday night, Andrea took her turn sleeping on a cot in

Thomas's room, while Sean went back to the hotel and slept in the bed there. Luckily, even though Thomas's room was a two-patient room, there was no other patient there during his stay. That made it nice. The cot was actually quite comfortable with a mattress on it and Andrea's own comforter from home. She thought ahead on that one too.

Since they had only brought one vehicle, Andrea went to the hotel Monday morning and brought Sean back to the hospital so they could spend the day there. It was quite a long, boring day. They took turns rocking Thomas in the chair while the other switched TV channels, heading back to the cafeteria for each meal. It was nice to give Thomas all of his feedings and have him much more alert. Andrea was so excited when she got him to smile for the first time after surgery. He was just as precious as could be. He was starting to get back his happy personality again.

Monday night, Sean went back to the hotel again, and Andrea stayed in the room with Thomas. They were told by the doctor that Thomas would be going home on Tuesday. What a short stay after open-heart surgery! They could not believe it. Four nights in the hospital and he was going home. Andrea had tons of packing to do with all of the stuff she had brought for bedding for Thomas's crib and comforters for her own bed. She spent time taking numerous trips down to pack the car before they had Thomas officially discharged from Emanuel Hospital for the second time in his short life.

The last thing the doctor needed to do was take out the drain tube. Thomas had two tiny little holes at the base of his sternum with tubes coming out of them, which drained excess blood from his body cavity. They pulled out the tubes, which were surprisingly long. There were strings that were previously sutured in place that were used to tie off and close those small openings in Thomas's chest.

expect a miracle  *189*

Andrea was afraid of putting Thomas in his car seat. She realized car seats were pretty constrictive, and she didn't want to apply any pressure to his sensitive rib cage. She put a small blanket that he had come out of surgery with, one that the hospital had given him, in between his sternum and the seatbelt so it would provide even the slightest bit of cushion for him just in case there was a sudden stop or braking.

That week, Andrea went back to work while Sean stayed home with Thomas. The following week they traded, and Andrea stayed home through Wednesday. Then they would all return to work and daycare. The daycare provider was afraid of taking him back so soon after open-heart surgery, and Andrea could tell she was concerned and attempted to calm her fears by telling her that Thomas was doing absolutely great.

### HEBREWS 12:1 NIV

Therefore, since we are surrounded by such a great cloud of witnesses, let us throw off everything that hinders and the sin that so easily entangles, and let us run with perseverance the race marked out for us.

During the month of March, Andrea's co-worker, Patty, told her about an organization called the Sparrow Clubs. She introduced Andrea to a lady named Karen, who was one of the representatives for the club. Sparrow Clubs was an organization that got businesses to sponsor children and got kids in schools together to do community service and earn money for it. The children would turn in hours they earned doing their community service and the company sponsor would pay Sparrow Clubs the amount those children had earned. The children could also go above and beyond and do fundraisers and raise extra money for their Sparrow child. Andrea filled out an application that basically laid out Thomas's situation and Sean and Andrea's humongous list of medical bills. Their total bill at the end of everything, after the entire pregnancy and all surgeries, was over $380,000! The awesome thing was Andrea had super insurance that covered her hospital stay and her surgeries. They did pay a substantial portion out of their own pockets, of course, for travel and out-of-pocket deductibles.

For whatever reason, they had decided to cover Thomas under Sean's insurance, which turned out to be a big mistake. They should have left him under the insurance that paid so well for Andrea. They ended up struggling and fighting with that insurance company to get them to pay the bills that were coming through. The total amount out-of-pocket that Sean and Andrea needed to pay was about $20,000, not bad considering a total bill of nearly $400,000!

Sparrow Clubs and the experience it created for Sean and Andrea was such a wonderful thing. Not only did it help them pay their bills, but it made them realize that, although they thought they could do everything in life on their own, everybody at one point in their lives is going to need help. Sean and Andrea were in a place where they wanted to be self sufficient and thought they could be. It was an excellent experience to be forced to face the reality they couldn't do it on their own. They had to rely on other people for help.

Help came from strangers and, best of all, friends. Andrea's parents put a check for $1,000 into her birthday card. Her grandparents mailed her a check for $1,000. When she gave John a check for nearly $1,000 to pay him back for paying for her insurance while she was technically unemployed, he voided it and gave it back to her. The gesture made her cry at her desk in disbelief. Karla and her children also raised $350 for them. The most wonderful part of it all was when Andrea mailed the last check for $800 to the heart surgeon's office. His final bill was paid, in full, two weeks before Thomas's first birthday. God

**expect a miracle** *191*

had provided them with everything they needed but not more than they needed. That was another lesson they learned. He will provide.

They very gradually settled into what would be considered a normal life. Going to work day in and day out. Dropping Thomas off at day care day in and day out. It was nice, and Andrea liked the routine. At one point, Thomas had an accident at daycare, and Andrea got a call from the provider, who said he had been hit in the face and his teeth were bleeding. Andrea's perspective on it was a little bit different than she would have expected. She was upset about it, of course, but after the dust settled, she thought to herself, *These are the things normal parents deal with. Children get injuries. Someday he'll probably break a bone. These are the things I was expecting to happen. These are normal.* And it actually made her happy to experience the normal troubles of childhood that Thomas would go through.

**1 CORINTHIANS 2:9 NIV**
No eye has seen, no ear has heard, no mind has conceived
what God has prepared for those who love him.

It will take Sean and Andrea a lifetime to absorb all of the lessons they learned through their experiences; the rest of their lives to consider the impact it had in shaping who they would become. The emotional burden, the excitement, the stress, and the strain on a marriage, the financial pressure, the family burdens, and the individual personality changes they each went through. Also, the lessons Andrea faced at being in San Francisco by herself, and lessons Sean faced at having the burden at home by himself. They knew their experiences were going to help them help other people, and that is the ultimate goal. The ultimate goal is to turn hardship into a help to others. There is no lasting damage done to Thomas. He will grow up knowing he had a very rough, but special and miraculous beginning.

Andrea started getting excited about the experiences, thinking what a wonderful blessing they would turn out to be if she could use them to share this miraculous message from God, of how He is still working in people's lives today. Not just when He was here on earth, but still day in and day out, working miracles. Her excitement turned into taking the journal she had written and turning it into a book. Sean and Andrea know there is so much more to Thomas's story and Thomas's life than what happened in those two years. The lessons they'll take with them are innumerable, and the lessons they will help other people learn are exciting to ponder. The opportunities it will create, the future it will give to other parents and other children to hear Thomas's story and to know these things did happen and that things can turn out alright in the end.

After working with Andrea for four years, John would look at her sometimes and say, "I cannot believe the person you have become."

Andrea looked at him and said, "It's all Thomas. I love being a mom."

John said, "It's not that. There's more to you. There's more to your personality, and it's all changed for the better."

John was not a believing person. He didn't spend any time thinking about God. He told Andrea that, on the Friday morning before Thomas's heart surgery, he stood outside and looked up at the sky and said a prayer to God, "You take care of that little boy."

Thomas was already using his circumstances to witness to people, and he didn't even know it yet.

### 1 PETER 1:6–7 NIV

In this you greatly rejoice, though now for a little while you may

> have had to suffer grief in all kinds of trials. These have come
> so that your faith—of greater worth than gold, which perished
> even though refined by fire—may be proved genuine and may
> result in praise, glory and honor when Jesus Christ is revealed.

Andrea thinks back to the day she went shopping in Portland with Mary and April, when she was standing in the corner of the music box shop, seemingly all alone. The inscription on that music box spoke directly to her from God. She carried that message with her through all of the experiences. Through the whole time in San Francisco, all of the tests, every ultrasound, every surgery, she kept it in her mind. She kept it in her heart. Although she was very scared, deep down in her soul, she always felt like Thomas would be okay. She didn't want to admit it to herself *just in case*, but she always felt Thomas would end up fine. She was basically being told by the message on the music box to be aware of what was happening around her. Be aware of what was happening within her and to watch ... and wait ... and listen, and to do exactly what that music box said, which was ... *expect a miracle*.

# Personal Note from the Author

There are times I've felt so alone in my experience. Sure, I might meet someone, somewhere, who could relate to one or two separate events, but not certain moments, and definitely not the experience as a whole. I will probably never meet another person who can relate to our extreme situations. I had to come to grips with the fact that my situation is unique to me. Even Sean, who went through the whole thing with me, didn't have the same experience I had. He felt different emotions at different times than I did. We went through the same thing but from our own perspectives and with our own strengths and weaknesses.

You may have a situation that you've faced, or are currently facing, that makes you feel like you are completely alone. It could be something like divorce, death of a loved one, addiction of any sort, (addictions come in many shapes and sizes), loss of a job, medical concerns. I'm sure you could find a self-help book at any store that would offer you one hundred ways to deal with your problems or heal your physical pain or emotional baggage all on your own; or there is probably a support group out there where you can find strength in people who have shared in your pain. I'm sure there are benefits from some self-help books, and I believe that support groups are an important way for us to help each other through this life, but we will never be the right source of help for each other in the long run.

There is only One source of help that is always available to you. One source that is waiting with baited breath to hear your call. One source that has the ability to turn your tears of sorrow into tears of joy. One source that has all the answers you've searched for ... *Why me? What do I do next? Where am I going? How will I get through this? Why did I have that bad thing happen to me?* That source is Jesus Christ. My strength to endure a long struggle came from the knowledge I have that Jesus is in control of my life. How do I know that's true and not just hot air? Because I chose to give Him control of my life. Once you do that, once you give up control, you give up trying to take care of everything by yourself. You also give up the stress, the emotional pain, and the heartache of regret.

Life without Jesus is like mountain climbing without a harness. It's exciting and fun, but dangerous, and will eventually end in your demise. Having Jesus in your life is like having all the fun of mountain climbing with all the safety of a rope and harness.

I know we've all heard of Jesus, but who is he really? Jesus is the Son of God. God, the father, did the unthinkable and sacrificed his only son to save all of us. Jesus came and lived a sinless life on this earth to die for our sins. Why? Because he's the only One who could live a sinless life and be worthy of offering himself as a perfect sacrifice for sin. No one likes to hear that they are a sinner, but ya know, we all are. Every one of us is a sinner.

Sin is anything that you do that separates you from God. There is definite right and wrong in this world; all things are not relative. Our society tells us that what works for you is okay for you, but not for me, but it's all good. No. Don't buy into that. That is the easiest way to justify sin in our lives. God

*196* andrea merkord

gave us the Bible so that we would know what was right and wrong.

Romans 6:23 says, "For the wages of sin is death, but the gift of God is eternal life in Christ Jesus our Lord."

Romans 5:8 says, "But God demonstrated his own love for us in this: while we were yet sinners, Christ died for us."

Okay, so Jesus Christ died for my sins. If I believe that, what do I do about it? The good news is that there is nothing God expects from you that would help you to *earn* your way to heaven. All you need to do is invite Jesus into your life by admitting you believe in Him. I'm going to show you a sample prayer, and if you believe in Jesus, you just pray it. If you want to give up the pain and the fear, the feeling of being all alone, then you can ask Jesus to take control of your life by praying this prayer.

Dear God,

Thank you for sending Jesus to die for my sins. Thank you that Jesus was raised from the dead so that I could have eternal life in heaven. I invite Jesus into my life right now and accept his gift of forgiveness and eternal life. Thank you that I am now your child. Please take control of my life and help me to become the kind of person you want me to be.

In Jesus' name, Amen.

Welcome into the family of Christ. Now, go find someone close to you and tell them what an exciting decision you just made. The best is still to come!

expect a miracle  *197*

1   University of Maryland Medicine. www.umm.edu
2   http://www.tttsfoundation.org. June, 2006.